HEALTHY THROUGH HODGKIN'S

How one woman combined conventional medicine with natural methods to cure her cancer and support her body.

KYLENE TERHUNE

outskirts
press

This book is dedicated to every person diagnosed with Hodgkin's. YOU are a warrior. I hope this book brings encouragement to you as you put on the armor to fight this battle.

And to my sweet, kind and loving husband who has supported me before, during and after cancer and encouraged me every step of the way. I love you.

Table of Contents

Foreword

It was just another day of scrolling through social media. That was until I came across a post in a group of cutting-edge healthcare practitioners. The post said, "Is there such a thing as a functional medicine oncologist? If so, can you share below? And any cancer/lymphoma resources out there, I would love to hear about that as well! (books, podcasts, physicians) Thanks!"

Kylene posted this request after newly finding out about her own Hodgkin's Lymphoma Diagnosis. I replied right away because, as it turns out, there is such a thing as a Functional Medicine Oncologist. Technically, I am board certified in Naturopathic Oncology.

As a Naturopathic Oncologist, I support people every day with their cancer. Most of the time that means integrating natural therapies into conventional treatments (like chemo and radiation) to reduce side effects and keep people healthy, functioning, and sometimes even experience their best health in years.

When Kylene and I hopped on the phone, there was an instant connection. But I could tell she was thrown by a Naturopathic Doctor supporting the use of chemotherapy. The thing is, only 15 years earlier, I was in a similar position to Kylene. My partner, Phil, was diagnosed with Lymphoma when we were just 25 years old. I knew the stats. I also knew that we could get her through chemo treatment healthy and strong.

During our calls, I was so impressed by Kylene's knowledge of health, supplements, labs, and diet. I couldn't help but think...she knows so much already, why does she need me?

Kylene always asked such amazing questions and came to our appointments with research and ideas. I love working with people that are passionate about health and take health care into their own hands, which made visits with Kylene a favorite part of the day. As treatments progressed, it became clear the expertise I brought to the table, but it was also clear that Kylene wasn't learning just for herself.

Kylene has been on a quest to learn about optimizing health since 2015. She has been a functional health coach, podcast host, and overall healthy living inspiration for many people (Including me! I love her live videos).

When Kylene was diagnosed with Lymphoma, she took the years of reading functional lab work and health coaching and applied it to her own life. Always wanting to give back and educate others based on what she has learned in her own life, Kylene started taking notes about her Hodgkin's Lymphoma journey. What worked, what didn't, and what was missing.

One of the things missing? An amazing Hodgkin's Lymphoma book that helped people to get through treatment and stay healthy during and after cancer treatment. I wish that this resource was available to Phil and me 15 years ago. But I am so grateful that this book is available for you NOW.

Kylene, thank you for sharing your Hodgkin's experience with us all. Thank you for being an inspiration. Thank you for always taking what you learn and sharing it with others. I am so grateful that I got to know you during this time of your life. I can't wait for whoever needs this book right now to get to know you too. I know they will learn that you are kind, spunky, and full of practical tips and resources.

Love,
Dr. Heather Paulson, ND, FABNO

My dream for this book is to be placed into the hands of any woman diagnosed with Hodgkin's disease (also known as Hodgkin lymphoma). You can read it front to back to get a big picture (and to get to know me!), or you can skip to certain chapters that look particularly interesting, although most build on each other. There is also a resource chapter in the back that you can mark up or highlight if anything catches your eye while reading that you want to come back to later. That chapter is there for you to use before, during, or after treatment depending on what you need. There are additional resources in there for those with breast cancer or other cancers because anyone that reads this book knows SOMEONE with cancer, and now you have resources to provide to them.

I want you to read this book as if we are friends hanging out in my kitchen drinking some mushroom coffee together (Foursigmatic is my favorite!). I am not a medical doctor, licensed dietitian, naturopath or degreed nutritionist so this book should not be read as though I am. I am a functional health coach who is obsessed with health information, loves researching, loves helping others find the path to optimal health, and loves how food can build up and nourish our bodies when used appropriately. And well... I also happened to get diagnosed with Hodgkin's. To me (looking back of course—not when it happened) this was another opportunity to learn more about something I never would have researched on my own. But now that I have, I want to take my nerdy health obsession and use it to help anyone diagnosed with this to navigate their healing journey in a way that allows them to make educated choices, feel comfortable in their care, and know that they have options. I want you to be able to support your body to feel as strong as possible during treatment. Emotionally *and* physically.

This book is not intended to diagnose, treat or prevent any medical conditions, and it is not meant to replace medical advice. Please keep your oncologist or doctor apprised of any changes you wish to make or include with your care and discuss your options with a professional.

So grab a fluffy blanket and let's get started!

1

My Story

HELLO FRIEND. THAT'S how I view you reading this book. By the end I hope we will be friends. Going into this journey I had no idea what to expect, but writing this book to encourage you as you embark on this massive and stormy journey is worth it if it can give you a few laughs and perhaps a few tips along the way to make the ride a bit smoother for you.

As I write this chapter, I am sitting on a flight from Chicago to Los Angeles. While I am really excited to be making this business trip to meet some awesome entrepreneurial women, gain some valuable information on how to grow my business, and soak up some sun, I can't stop thinking about three words: I have cancer.

This is actually the 2nd or 3rd book I've sat down to write over the past few years. One of them was an autobiography (because who doesn't want to know everything about my life?!) and another was all about how to stop dieting and discover your #YOUtrition which ended up becoming my 6-week online program and never a book... and this one, well, this one is completely unplanned. Honestly, I never knew if this would even be published. I thought it may end up simply being a cathartic journal. But I chose to document my journey through video and this book because there is so much to this experience that is scary, unknown, and new. There is so much of your life that dramatically changes when you first get diagnosed and until it happens to you, you simply don't understand what others who have already fought the battle have gone through.

Cancer is an extremely emotional experience. In fact, about an hour ago, I was in the airport bathroom in between flights crying my eyes out. I tried to contain myself on the plane, I really did. But as we were pulling up to the gate the tears insisted on spilling down my cheeks, one after the other until my nose started getting stuffy, my face got red, and if anyone near me had any observation skills there was no hiding my silent meltdown.

I'm writing this not to ask for pity, but to share a part of this disease that I never knew about. We always hear or see the "strong" moments right? Social media allows us to pick and choose our highlight reel, and often, I think, those with cancer stay to themselves, pull away from social media, and instead reach out to those closest to them. Others who want to be a beacon, a light, an encouragement, choose to stay active on social media, embrace a positive attitude and utilize it to lift others up and be a positive example of fighting through the rough times. There's nothing wrong with either approach. But in both instances we often miss the tears, the silent meltdowns (and the not-so silent) and the fall into your husband's arms, full-on breakdowns.

For me, I fall somewhere in the middle of wanting to share it all and wanting to disappear. I love social media. I've met new friends, found clients (that often become friends) and networked with some incredible professionals. So when I realized that I would be going down this road, it only seemed natural for me to share it openly and honestly. The good and the bad. Sometimes I seem perky and energetic and other times I have cried on video, live, for everyone to see. The thing about that is that both of those are really me. Those are both completely honest depictions of how I feel in that very moment and truth be told, I can't tell how any day will go, even at this point.

But let me start at the beginning. Hi, my name is Kylene Terhune. I'm a Functional Diagnostic Nutrition Practitioner who, over the past three years, has healed my gut, worked on balancing my hormones, and improved my overall health along with the health of family, friends, and many personal clients. But now I have cancer. Nodular Sclerosis Hodgkin Lymphoma, Stage 1A, non-bulky to be exact. Yup! I'm extremely healthy. My blood markers are good, and my health has actually *improved* in many ways over the past several years. But I have cancer.

December 25th, 2018, I was sitting at my parent's table for Christmas breakfast when I said:

"Hey mom, look at this lump I found in my neck."

"Oh Ky, you better get that checked out."

"Yeah I know, I will."

"Maybe it's just a lymph node. Have you been sick?"

"Yeah maybe, that's sort of what we were thinking. I've had a little drainage. Not enough to cause a large lump though and normally your neck would be all sore and stuff..."

A few weeks earlier I had noticed a lump by my right clavicle. I can't remember the exact day, and I can't remember how I found it. I obviously didn't think much of it at the time, but something made me mention it to my husband Patrick. After his and my mom's concern at Christmas I became a little more worried about it, so I began Googling of course, and that's never helpful. All the outcomes were dreary and of course there was the C word. If you have a painless lymph node in your neck it may be... cancer.

So I set an appointment to see my general MD but I chose to see a new doctor. I hardly ever go to the doctor and we had been thinking of finding a new one anyway, so I felt like this was a good opportunity to "try a new one out".

Once I felt the lump, and began noticing it more, I discovered that I could do a fun little trick with it. Some days I would see it and some days I would think "oh wow, it's definitely gone down!" Until I realized that no, I could roll my shoulder back and turn my head a certain way and *boom* there it as. A lump the size of a ping-pong ball popping out of the right side of my neck.

We met with the new doctor on January 11th. She asked me a lot of questions, and I felt great that day. I was sure this was nothing (mostly) and we left with an order for routine bloodwork and an ultrasound to look at the lump.

On January 15th I had the ultrasound and it was a piece of cake. I went in, showed the ultrasound tech my neat trick, popping the lump out so she could see it, laughing together and then laying down so she could plop the ultrasound goop on my neck and do her thang. A few minutes later I was cleaned up and out the door. Later that day, I received a call from the doctor's office letting me know that the ultrasound was inconclusive. They had been looking to see if they could confirm a liquid or a solid mass. If it was liquid then it could be something harmless like a cyst. If it was solid, well, that would lead to more tests.

Since the ultrasound was inconclusive she recommended a CT (computed tomography) scan with contrast. I didn't know what contrast was so I looked it up; turns out it's this yucky iodine concoction that helps your organs to be more visible in the scan. So on January 25th I went in for the CT scan. A very nice nurse talked me through the procedure and let me ask as many questions as

I wanted. By the way, I totally thought a CT scan was a big long tube machine. It's not, it's the shape of a donut, so don't worry, you aren't completely closed in; within a foot or two you could be on one side or the other. You lay down and get pushed through the donut to whatever area they want to scan, and you get moved around a little while it takes pictures. The nice CT tech hooked me up to the contrast IV where the contrast solution would be pumped into my bloodstream, explained that it would probably feel a little funny and that I may notice it in my throat before it rushes down to my groin where I would feel like I peed my pants. "You won't" she reassured me, giggling.

She was right—whoa the contrast felt bizarre in the back of my neck as it went in. Not painful or anything, just weird. Then BOOM! right down to my groin and a few seconds later WOOSH it was gone. Once we were done I commented on how fast it went away and she said "oh yeah! That's how fast your blood circulates! It's already filtering through your kidneys and on its way to your bladder!" Aren't our bodies super cool? Besides a slight numb feeling in the back of my throat I felt normal and was soon on my way back home.

A few hours later I was sitting in a meeting when I got a call from my doctor. Phones are so super cool now; when you get a voicemail you can also see the transcript and sort-of cheat to see if the call is important. I saw that it was my doctor calling, and suddenly I couldn't wait for the meeting to be over. It's never good when it's your actual doctor and not a nurse. So I rushed out of the meeting, got in my car and called her back while sitting in the parking lot.

"Your CT scan showed a mass that was 5.8 by 3.1 centimeters. It's possible that this is lymphoma and that's why I called you personally. You have two options right now. You can get it biopsied or you can go the route of surgery where you get it removed and biopsied at the same time. Just let me know what you'd like to do."

OMG. WHAT?! "Ok um, let me think about it. I'll talk to my husband and call you back."

So I immediately called Patrick and asked him what he thought we should do... He asked better questions than I did, so I said; "Hey, let's get on a three-way call so you can ask the questions and we can talk to her together."

Boy, was I not ready for that second call. I was sort of fine the first time; the doctor seemed not sure and I wasn't too alarmed. But when we called back, she used the cancer word a lot, noted that there were other lymph nodes in the area that seemed a little swollen, and told us that the CT report said that it's likely lymphoma, and less likely that it's something like a hematoma or cyst.

Wow. "Ok let's get a biopsy then." So she set it up and we got off the phone. Almost immediately I started crying. Cancer? What?! No way. There is NO WAY this is actually becoming a thing. How the heck did this happen? The past few years I've been getting *healthier* not grow-ing a tumor!

The next few hours were filled with phone call after phone call after phone call.

"Mom... ... [excessively long pause]"

"Ky, what is it?"

[tears] "She said she found a mass..."

After that I called my friend who is a nutritionist and chiropractor and that phone call helped me make sense of it all. He was encouraging, he was frustrated that she used the cancer word so soon without a biopsy, and he encouraged me that it's possible to go the route of sur-gery and biopsy at the same time to avoid cancer seeding. Yes, I looked it up. It's totally possible. Cancer seeding is when you get a biopsy and it disrupts cancer cells releasing them into your lymph and/or blood stream increasing the likelihood (although low) of spreading your cancer to other areas of your body.

Holy crap! Ok surgery it is. Now this was a Friday (have you noticed how dramatic news seems to come on Fridays?) so we had all weekend before we could do anything. Turns out, God was probably in that too. I had called to schedule my biopsy after the hubbub of phone calls in the parking lot, but they were already out of office so I would have had to call back Monday anyway. This meant that we had all weekend to worry and stew, wonder and think before being able to do anything.

So Monday rolls around, and after doing some research and thinking on my friend's advice, I call back my MD and ask for a surgeon referral instead. As we prepared to go to the surgeon we had all these other questions like: "How long would recovery be? Would this affect the use of my arm?" Etc. etc. etc.... I sort of assumed surgery was a done deal. Bing bang boom. Let's get this sucker out and biopsy it and be done.

January 30th Patrick and I walked into the surgeon's office with a list of questions ready to go. I was sitting in the patient room, more nervous than I expected. I *felt* mentally calm, yet my body was betraying me as I was sweating through my shirt and gripping my phone to make sure I didn't forget to access my list of prepared questions once we got rolling.

After waiting nervously for a while the doctor walked in and I was pleasantly surprised. Nice, happy, communicative and willing to answer questions, I was really bummed when he then said he couldn't be my surgeon. But let's back up. After checking the lump on my neck and looking at my CT and ultrasound, he explained that it was in a very difficult place to operate. He told me that the lump was very near several nerves controlling my arm, by some pretty major muscles, and turns out, it's right next to the top of my right lung too. He recommended that I go for a biopsy first and even if we go for surgery, he would rather send me to a specialist neck surgeon.

Well, that wasn't great. But it wasn't bad either. He actually gave us quite a bit of hope that it could be so many things. He didn't rush to lymphoma, and so neither did we. After that, I got a little annoyed at my MD for jumping to lymphoma and using the cancer word so quickly. It could be anything right?! Why would you say that without definitive proof?

So the next stage was to schedule an appointment with the specialist neck surgeon. I thought, hey, maybe this specialist will have a different opinion. Maybe it's a tricky surgery, but as a specialist he does things like this all the time and has super-fancy, cool surgery tools that make this doable. February 6th rolled around and I had an appointment with a surgeon who specializes in ENT (ears, nose and throat). I was less nervous this time, but still came armed with my phone full of questions. This surgeon repeated the same thing that the first one did. "This is a really tricky spot. There are a lot of nerves here, some that control your arm, some control your vocal cords..."

Hold up. My vocal cords? For those of you who don't know me, my undergraduate degree was in vocal performance. That's right. Opera. No way Jose. Don't mess with my vocal cords! Anyway, all the rest of the advice still applied. It's near my lung, he wouldn't recommend surgery, go get a biopsy.

With our surgery options exhausted we said ok to the biopsy. The nice thing was that now that we were in specialist-land, the ENT guy also referred us to a biopsy specialist. This is always nice because things move more quickly than in hospital settings. I was in the ENT's office Wednesday and in the pathologist's office Friday so pretty quick. Like I said, all the bad news comes on Fridays.

One thing you should know about me. I don't really like needles. So much so that when I was a kid, I had several cavities, which turned into several fillings, which of course meant several shots of Novocain. I hated those huge shots that pinched SO much that eventually I asked to have any future cavities drilled and filled without numbing shots. Yup. That's right, put that in my chart and don't you forget it. Bonus, they are way more careful when they know you can feel everything. And by the way, I never regretted that decision. Occasionally, some cold air would hit a nerve and that would hurt a tiny bit, but overall, little-to-no pain and totally worth the lack of shots in my opinion.

So, you can imagine how I felt when I realized I would have to have a biopsy to figure out what this thing in my neck was. I was not excited about it. I mean, we all know what a biopsy is right? HUGE needles going into your (in my case) NECK to diagnose the cells and tissue! Ok. Breathe. I know man, I know. It's scary. So there I was, February 8th, 2019, about to get a needle stuck into me. My sweet husband came with me for an 8:30am appointment. We filled out some forms and the nice nurse took us into a small doctor's office. The nice thing about being in private practice is the doc gets to choose the elevator music, so in this case, it was normal radio music and we laughed. I mean, come on, what else do you have to talk about while you are waiting for a man to come stab you in the neck?

The nurse came in and did her thing and then a few minutes later the pathologist came in. He was an unassuming man with glasses who seemed kind of quiet but you could tell right away his goal was to put you at ease. He let Patrick hold my hand and explained everything before he did it. Trying to distract me he asked if I had kids, and he talked about his daughter throughout the procedure. So let's talk about the procedure because even though you might know what a biopsy is, I certainly didn't *know* what a *biopsy is* if you know what I mean.

First, he gave me two large shots of lidocaine near my collarbone. That numbed me up pretty good. I laughed because even more than not liking needles, I *really* don't like the feeling of being numb. I remembered back in the dentist days how awful it felt to "feel" what was happening without well, *feeling* it. Turns out, this experience felt totally different. Go figure. The two shots of lidocaine ended up being the worst part. After I was good and numb, he went in for the biopsy. Here is where my descriptions get more vague because I had to look away. If you want details you can ask my hubby because he was watching the whooooooole thing. The two biopsies were completely painless. I really didn't feel a thing although I did freak out a little when I saw out of the corner of my eye that his hand was pumping up and down and up and down. Wow. That just seems violent. And super painful. Crap. Is this going to hurt later?

After those two biopsies were over, he took the cells he collected and went to another room to observe them under the microscope. Like I said, it's nice to be in specialist world. This guy would not only do the biopsy but give us a preliminary diagnosis before we left. Patrick ran to the restroom while this was happening, so when the doc came back and said "Let's wait for your husband" I had a horrible feeling that the talk wasn't going to go well.

"Well, um, it does look like it's Hodgkin lymphoma, so I'd like to take a core biopsy if that's ok with you," he said in his kind and shuffly way.

"Um ok, I guess. What does that mean?"

"That means we need to go into the actual tumor and grab some tissue so we can gather more information."

So back down on the table I went. I was still numb, so they proceeded right away. Apparently the core biopsy needle is much bigger but as my head was turned away of course, I didn't see it.

"There is a little popping sound with this one, so try not to jump ok?"

He inserted the needle into the tumor, there is a pop sound; I guess that's how it "grabs" the tissue. He did this twice as tears began to run down my cheeks, and then it was over.

Then, and this is a critical detail, he asked what kind of Band-Aid I wanted. "We have um, regular, or The Incredibles, or um, oh, we have Wonder Woman…"

"Wonder Woman obviously." I laughed.

The doctor looked through his microscope again and determined that, yes, it did look like Hodgkin's. He continued to explain what tests he was going to run with the core biopsy and what that meant, but honestly Patrick and I both zoned out at this point and didn't remember much after hearing the words, "It looks like Hodgkin's". The whole movie scenario where dramatic news is shared and everything fades into the background really happened. His lips were moving, and our heads were nodding, but nothing was really being absorbed.

"Please reach out to me with any questions. I really don't mind. I'll call you Monday with more information."

We left his office, walked to the car and immediately called my parents. I had Patrick start the call because I wasn't sure I could speak clearly without crying *again*. He explained everything and we decided to go get some coffee. Coffee dates are one of our favorite ways to spend time together and right now we had time and we needed to talk. So that's what we did. I was trying to think of all the positives, how God had timed this so that I was as healthy as I am, how I chose to see a new doctor who led us to the nicest pathologist in the world, how we are blessed and fortunate to have many resources financially and personally so that whatever came we would have connections and the ability to handle this. We knew that thinking this way would not be easy moving forward. But we also felt that there was a driving force and purpose behind this new part of our lives.

Looking back now, I realize I was in shock. This state of shock lasted for several months as the reality of my diagnosis began to sink in and we spent many hours researching and thinking and planning. Working in the functional medicine world, I naturally wanted to look into alternative treatments. So I watched a summit about alternative cancer treatment, I bought materials, I called facilities in and out of the country to get more information on their treatment, and I researched the heck out of my options. I reached out to a community of functional medicine practitioners and doctors and asked if there was such a thing as a functional oncologist. They pointed me in the direction of a naturopathic integrative oncologist in the community who specialized in integrative cancer care. Turns out her husband had also had Hodgkin's and is now cancer-free. So I reached out right away and got a call with her.

"Chemo is really effective for Hodgkin's, so I would recommend doing that. Over the next week they will probably…" And again I was in shock. An integrative oncologist who specializes in integrative treatment telling me that chemo is the way to go? At first I was almost angry. I expected other options. How could someone be telling me I needed chemo?!

But she wasn't the only person who told me this. Hodgkin's is unique in that the efficacy of chemotherapy is 95per cent which is almost unheard of in the cancer world. More times than not, chemo actually *does* work to put you into remission.

Patrick was researching too, and he came across the Cancer Treatment Centers of America (CTCA). What appealed to us was their willingness to use integrative approaches—they have naturopaths on staff and talk to you about diet changes based on the work of Patrick Quillin who wrote *Beating Cancer with Nutrition*. To clarify, the premise of the book is not to *treat* cancer with nutrition, but he shares how nutrients, foods and supplements can help you stay stronger, respond better and avoid side-effects during conventional treatments. We wanted to find out more.

We wanted a second opinion about potential treatment, and getting into the local oncologist for that proved to be a problem. The scheduling systems and communication processes were not smooth and it was difficult to get my initial appointment. So we flew out to the Chicago CTCA to speed things up. They paid for our flight, set us up in lodging, and scheduled all the tests and appointments for the few days we were there. Amazing; at last I was going to get answers.

While there I received a PET (positron emission tomography) scan for staging of the cancer, and another biopsy, but this time on my breast. I need to explain this... In the midst of all these cancer appointments I had scheduled a routine gynecologist appointment and she found lumps in both of my breasts. Since I had just been diagnosed with lymphoma, the red flags went up and everyone wanted to biopsy one of these lumps. I figured, let's get all the things done that we can in one trip, so we got the mammogram and the biopsy on my breast done at CTCA as well. Thankfully, the breast biopsy showed that the lump was benign.

A few days later, the CTCA oncologist met with me and let me know that I had stage 1A, non-bulky, nodular sclerosis Hodgkin lymphoma. I'll break it down for you:

Stage 1: There is only one tumor, or tumors in one quadrant of the body.

A: **No symptoms.**

Non-bulky: The tumor(s) are less than 10 cm.

The doctor recommended that I take three months of treatment, which meant six sessions of chemotherapy, no radiation, and assuming my follow up PET scan was clear, that would be it.

After he had explained his recommended course of treatment, he sat there and let me ask questions, and he and the nurses let me know what to expect should we decide to pursue treatment at CTCA.

We thanked them, came home, and set an appointment with my local oncologist. My goal was to see if she felt ok following this treatment plan because it seemed like the minimum treatment available and I certainly didn't want any more than was absolutely necessary! I also wanted to stay as near to home as possible since I had no way of anticipating how I might feel once treatments began.

The local oncologist met with me and said this was not the "standard of care" so she wanted to call the doctor from CTCA to ask that he show her the studies he was basing his recommendations on. She would then be more able to follow his recommendations. They connected, she agreed, and we got started.

The next step was to consider fertility preservation. Since chemotherapy can affect your future ability to have children and we had just begun getting more serious about starting our own family, we decided to take this step as a precaution. Once I got home, I scheduled an appointment with a fertility clinic that happened to be conveniently located a few miles down the road. Fertility preservation became a huge part of my life at this time, so I have devoted a large portion of chapter two to it – if you too, are in this situation, then please do read "Things you need to know...that I didn't". See you there...

I was diagnosed in February, and began treatment in May. Does that seem too long to you, or about right? For me, it was partially due to fertility preservation treatment, which took a whole month, not including recovery time, and partially due to the fact that I wanted to think, pray, research and feel good about whatever decision I ended up making.

I finally came to the decision that the best thing to do for me would be three months of conventional treatment, paired with the approach of the integrative oncologist I had reached out to. If I was going to go conventional, I was going to do everything in my power to protect my body through the process.

There were three primary reasons I decided on conventional treatment:

1. Other therapies would take me away from my home and family for weeks to months at a time. While there are clinics available in the U.S., many are out of the country, and all would require travel and stay at the facility.
2. If conventional treatment had a 95 per cent success rate for my specific cancer, I wanted equal assurances if I chose another route. I couldn't find it.
3. I really wanted to get this done. I was looking at three months vs potential years of slow progress using other treatment options.

It's not that I don't believe that there is something out there that can be just as effective as chemo; I just didn't find the information I needed that fulfilled *my* goals by the time I made the decision. So I chose an integrative, blended path.

Ultimately, treatment started on May 9th and ended on July 19th. Chemotherapy was done every other week on Fridays for three months. Ten days after my final treatment I got my follow-up PET scan, and one week after that my doctor let me know that the scan was clear. The mass (tumor) was still there and hadn't changed in size much, but the cancer was no longer active. I would still need ongoing monitoring of the tumor itself, but otherwise, I was good to go! I had made it through the treatment with only a few blips and no major symptoms and came out of it with no long-term symptoms or pain. Praise God!

Post-treatment has been its own journey. After receiving the PET results, when you think I might have been jumping for joy, I simply didn't know *how* to feel. It took me about a full day to really soak it in. After that, I wanted to get back to real life but it took me a hot minute to realize that I was still recovering. I had to learn how to balance getting back to normal with respecting my body as it healed.

Today, as I share this with you, I feel amazing and I have a life that I love. I know that you can too, and I hope that this book brings you encouragement, laughter, hope and information that you can take with you in this new chapter of life.

2

Things you need to know…
that I didn't

Take your time

WHEN I WAS about 20 years old, I met a guy. We started dating, I dropped out of school and within a year and a half we got married. There was something not right about the relationship and I felt it fairly early on. But every time I would break up with him he would manipulate me in to feeling like we should give it another go, convince me that he needed me blah blah blah… I remember crying on my honeymoon because I realized I had made huge mistake and I did NOT want to be married to this guy. I had hopped on the train and let it take me to a destination I did not want to be.

That's what a cancer diagnosis can feel like. And yes, I just compared my ex-marriage to cancer. Is anyone else giggling about that? Unfortunately, that was a cancer I allowed to happen and could have prevented it from developing at any time. It took the surgical removal of divorce to finally get that out of my life and move on.

With my clinical cancer diagnosis I wanted to take time to think about it. I wanted to feel like I was driving the speeding train of treatment and that I could change direction or even stop it whenever I wanted. I encourage you right now to stop, take a deep breath, and tell yourself out loud, "I am in charge." Because guess what - you *are*!

You have the power to research. To ask questions. To choose your treatment plan. To get a second or even a third opinion. To say no to extras. To be in control. Remember—this is YOUR body and YOUR life. You need to know what's happening and feel really good about the treatment plan. You need to have full confidence that what you choose will work so that you can go into it with the right mentality so that your emotions around the process encourage the healing to happen instead of discouraging it.

As I began this journey I thought: "How many people have I seen or known that have had cancer, yet I have *no* idea what they went through?" Then I began my flurry of doctor's visits and realized how many people are thrown into a system where they get a diagnosis, are told scary information, and thrown into treatment a week later! WOAH. That is *so fast*. Way too fast to make a life-altering decision. But we aren't really told that we have a choice.

My mission became about empowering women to become advocates for their own health and the health of their families and homes. One night I came up with the catchy phrase "Turning Homemakers into Healthmakers". Think about it... women are usually the decision-makers when it comes to health in our own bodies and in our homes. We most often do the grocery shopping, plan the meals, pack the lunches, choose the doctors... you get the picture. If cancer isn't enough of a jolt for you to take charge of your health long-term then I don't know what is! But I know I know...you're reading this book so I'm preaching to the choir! You *are* a healthmaker. You are here to do your research, get empowered, and make your own choices. Kudos to you my friend, you are amazing.

If you're reading this and you've already begun treatment, great! Maybe you already feel totally comfortable with that decision. We all do what we can, when we can, with the information we have. There are still plenty of options for you to take time and breathe and make sure you don't feel like others are driving the bus for you.

If you've picked up this book just before diagnosis, again, I would encourage you to take some time to breathe, pray, research and think through all the options. Here's a hot tip–if you are of reproductive age, take the next month to harvest your eggs and use that time to think things through–the doctors will totally support that decision!

Follow your gut

I was diagnosed at 32. My husband and I had been together for seven years and we had Keegan (my stepson who I call my son, and lives with us full time). I never had this major desire like many women to become a mother… ok scratch that… I had a major fear of pregnancy and giving birth. Let's just be honest. I didn't want to go through the pain and trash my body and well… you get it. But I did always want to adopt. So meeting this handsome Prince Charming who I fell madly in love with, and raising Keegan together, was the perfect situation for me. And then gradually (like, literally it took several years… and usually after a few cocktails) I began asking Patrick if he wanted more kids, if we should talk about it… what did he think?

I needed that warm-up time. I was priming my mind for the possibility. Getting myself mentally to the point where I knew I could do it and everything would be ok. I mean–that's what our female bodies are designed for right? As we discussed this over and over and over I came up with this secret little plan–get my body to a really healthy place and then get more serious.

I had already struggled for years with digestive stuff, hormone imbalances, fatigue... and knowing what I knew, and working as an FDN I wanted to have the perfect gut microbiome to grow a healthy baby if I chose to do so. I wanted my future "maybe-baby" to be set up for success! So while I had been working on, and improving, all these areas of my life and health, I wanted to get some really great test results back before moving forward with the baby-making.

So here we were, early 2019, just beginning to talk about the reality of trying for children of our own and *BAM*. I get this cancer diagnosis. Well, that put the kibosh on that didn't it? Because chemo can damage your ovaries and your fertility potential, we decided to go through the first phase of IVF (in-vitro fertilization) treatment and harvest as many eggs as we could... just in case.

Honestly, I felt pretty good during the hormone therapy—I was like woohoo—more hormones—I didn't feel too bad, and my little ovaries were responding well and doing their job like champs—growing healthy and massive eggs and keeping them there until harvest time. My body seemed to be all about it.

Everyone made retrieval sound like a cake walk. You go in, they suck out the eggs and you go home. No big deal. Um... no. That is *not* what happened. It *is* a big deal. And maybe it's because my ovaries were so obedient and pumped out 23 eggs (21 of which were viable) which is an insane amount (thank you healthy body!), but retrieval for me was a complete nightmare.

Wanna hear all about it? Keep reading. Not interested? Skip to the next subject header...

What was egg retrieval like?

Expensive, painful, and... dare I say it... not worth it? Ouch. I know that a lot of women out there live and breathe for the possibility of having children, but I haven't and honestly, had I known what all this would feel like *before* I signed up, I don't know if I would have followed through. However, everyone's body is different and many women have had better experiences that I did… So what's it like? Let me tell you:

Week 1 and Week 2

The first two weeks were easy. In fact, as I took my estrogen tablets (not recommended outside of this supervised and intentional process by the way) I felt pretty good! I generally have hormones on the low end of the range, so increasing my estrogen felt pretty good to me. The only side-effect I experienced was mild nausea that usually went away with a piece of gluten-free toast.

Week 3

Week three began the hormone shots; I used Gonal-F and Menopur which are a luteinizing hormone and a follicle-stimulating hormone. Basically, the goal is to get your follicles as big as possible so that during the retrieval process you harvest mature eggs that can then be used later. They will save *all* the eggs because they hope that as technology improves they may be able to mature the rest of the eggs someday as well.

Normally, your body matures about one follicle and releases one egg each month during ovulation… my body was maturing 24 follicles, the largest of which were about .75-.8 inches! As you can imagine, that meant that the ovaries began swelling. Even so, I wasn't terribly uncomfortable during this phase.

Every evening Patrick would give me two shots of those hormones in my belly and sometimes the jab hurt and sometimes there was a little soreness afterwards. But it was never horrible and always went away fairly quickly. Patrick felt much better being the administrator on the nights when they were pain free. Good job honey!

During this week you also have to do a blood draw and ultrasound every other day at the same clinic in order to monitor your follicle growth and estrogen levels so they can adjust your doses as necessary. This is all scheduled weeks in advance so you can plan accordingly.

Week 4

The beginning of this week (or potentially the end of week three) you start adjusting your shots. You begin taking a third shot that keeps your body from ovulating because *hello*, after three weeks of growing these follicles and thousands of dollars later, the last thing you want is to release all these suckers before harvest day!

Your ultrasounds and blood monitoring continue until they determine which day (out of a three-day range) your harvest will be. Then, 36 hours prior to your surgery time, you take a "trigger" shot. My harvest time was 7:30am on a Friday morning so my trigger shot was 7:30pm on the Wednesday. The day in between, no shots!

Retrieval day

Finally, it was retrieval day. I didn't know what to expect and was a bit nervous. I had an oops moment on the morning of surgery which almost threw the whole thing off. I drank water! I had only written down "no food" from midnight on, but apparently it was no food *or* water and they were pretty upset with me... this is because you can spit it up a bit when you are put under for the procedure... which, apparently I did a little. But since everything is time-sensitive, I agreed to the risks and we proceeded. So top tip, don't drink water before an operation, and double check if you are not sure.

When I woke up, I was not happy; I was in so much pain. Normally, when you wake up from something like this you feel all loopy, and happily hopped up on some legit pain meds… but no, I was hurting the moment I came to consciousness, and I was *not* ok with it.

For some reason, they could not administer intravenous pain killers or give me any at the clinic. So I walked out of that clinic with a pain prescription, loopy, and doubled over. I was probably freaking everyone out that was still in the waiting area!

On the plus side, we retrieved 23 eggs, which as I've done my research, seems to be a high amount. I got the impression that since I went through this process as a preservation thing and not since I was infertile to begin with, that I had a stronger "output" and my body participated more easily.

Unfortunately, I think because the output was so high, the pain was also… I had 23 eggs growing and the smallest of the follicles may be around .5 inches. In ovaries that are usually the size of your thumb, that's a lot of stretching to fit them all in! Then to have a hollow needle shoved up your hoo-ha to retrieve them all… well, inflammation followed.

The recovery

When I got home that morning, (Friday, April 12th) I was in excruciating pain. The whole procedure hadn't taken long and we were home before 10am. The pain was transferring beyond my ovaries and into other parts of my body (this is known as "referred" pain) like my back and I was convinced I was having kidney problems. Patrick ran to get the pain prescription and the first half of the day we were a bit behind the curve. I tried to take two and wait the full four hours, but then I ended up throwing up and in excruciating pain again before the next round sunk in. After that, I took smaller doses (one tablet instead of two) but more frequently so that the pain medication stayed in my system. Once we figured that system out, I felt ok after about 2:30pm and the rest of the day was spent sleeping and watching Netflix.

I was told to expect a little bit of pain, like period pain, on the day of retrieval, and then over the next three days start going back to normal. I think I had a stronger reaction than usual because day one was complete and utter misery.

Day two and three were better only in the sense that the excruciating pain was gone and I didn't have to live in bed.

I had extreme bloating throughout my abdomen making it difficult to eat regular food (Am I hungry? Am I not hungry? The pressure was messing everything up). I was mostly eating gluten-free bread or crackers, bone broth and chocolate pudding.

In addition to the pressure and swelling in my abdomen, I had pain and aches throughout my lower abdomen as well. Imagine wearing a belt of pain filled with rocks that shift around... that's sort of what it felt like. Walking was doable, but was also difficult. Getting up in bed or folding forward in any way was uncomfortable. Going to the bathroom was a whole other story... squeezing your abdomen to urinate becomes an unpleasant experience and you will most likely become constipated because of all the hormones and pain medication so there's an additional source of pressure and discomfort in the very area you don't want it!

I would highly recommend drinking plenty of water and taking a natural laxative like Senokot the day before surgery because those little things make a huge difference during recovery. I wish I had!

On day three I did a water enema in addition to the Senokot I had been using because I really needed that to be taken care of. I am used to doing coffee enemas, so I knew what to do. If you have never done one before, this may not be the time to start, but talk with a professional first if you do want to try it.

Occasionally it was also difficult to breathe from all the swelling and pressure in your abdominal area, so you may need to adjust to take deep breaths, and try not to breathe too far down into your diaphragm where all the inflammation is for a few days.

Day 4: Finally I hit a turning point! I experienced less bloating and the level of discomfort began to go down. I didn't mention it earlier, but during the tail end of the hormone treatments and on through the egg retrieval process, the scale began to creep up. It hit a high point a few days after the retrieval because of inflammation and water retention but for me, on day four, it began to go back down... yay! I was hoping that meant that the bloating, inflammation and the scale would continue to go down from here on!

By the end of the week there was still bloating and discomfort, but much more manageable than any of the days prior. I was also back to eating normally.

The results

As I mentioned, they successfully retrieved 23 eggs, and 21 of them were mature. I believe that if I need to pursue IVF treatment in the future, the worst is definitely behind me. Is it worth it? Like I said, I'm not sure. There's nothing I can do about it now, but I certainly didn't expect to be an invalid for three to four days post-retrieval and experience the level of discomfort I did. I knew that chemo would bring with it pain and side effects, so if I had known fertility preservation would be so painful too, would I have chosen it? Not sure. But I did, and now we have a safety net which is a good thing.

I wanted to share this because when I was researching what to expect there aren't a lot of stories sharing the aftercare experience. Perhaps I'm a special flower that just really experienced the max levels of pain and that's unusual, but if it's not, and you choose to go this route, I want you to be fully prepared. Because if having children is your dream, it's only a few days and you can definitely do it. If it's *not*, well now you know.

Should you choose to go through fertility treatments, here are some top tips from my experience:

1. Eat a healthy diet. There was one week where I really craved more carbs and sugar but other than that I stuck to my usual nutrition! Focus on veggies, water and healthy fats to support your fertility process.

2. Are you on the fence about fertility treatment? There are lots of other things to try first including changing your diet and lifestyle to improve your chances of conception. In fact, several of my personal clients have "accidentally" become pregnant after working together when previously it had been more difficult. Personally, had cancer not forced my hand, I wouldn't have chosen this for myself. I spent several years working on my hormones and balancing them naturally; I even eliminated my PMS completely and regulated my cycle to 28 days! There are lots of books and resources out there so I wouldn't recommend IVF as your first step to fertility, but sometimes it's a necessary step, so don't let yourself feel guilty if it is something you need to go through either.

3. Consider supplements. Curcumin, fish oil, multi-vitamins and probiotics are beneficial almost always, but certainly when you are trying to keep your inflammation low and your digestion regular. I was really happy that I didn't experience a lot of discomfort before the procedure. My healthcare team kept indicating that I would, but I didn't. I believe my diet helped me in this.

4. Drink plenty of water as soon as you begin to take the medicines. When I started taking the shots I didn't realize you could get dehydrated and I got behind at first. Staying up on your water intake really helps–be proactive!

5. Be aware of the reality of constipation. It's not helpful and it's not fun. Consider starting the day before retrieval with a natural laxative and get as much water as possible prior to the surgery cut off/ fasting time.

6. Regardless of how natural or healthy you are, do NOT shy away from the real pain medications if you need them. They exist for times like this and will help you get through the first 24-48 hours.

7. Remember: You *can* do this. Your body is designed to do amazing things, and it will recover and heal, and you can always assist it in detoxing this process as well.

8. Ask a family member or friend to make dinner the night of the surgery. You may be drinking liquids and downing bone broth, but it's extra helpful for your family to have some extra food that you don't have to stress about.

9. And finally, when you are taking lots of NSAIDS or pain RXs, consider taking some supplements to protect your tummy and gut lining. I got a little behind on this on day one and could tell that my tummy wasn't happy about it. Since then, I used GI Response which is a powder supplement you blend with water that contains L Glutamine which repairs your digestive lining, in addition to other herbs like slippery elm and marshmallow root that help soothe and heal as well.

Following retrieval

After retrieval, my oncologist and fertility specialists recommended a plan to get a shot to shut down my hormones and put me in menopause during treatment. The reasoning behind this is mainly two-fold:

1. Without cycling, they hope to keep you from losing extra blood during treatment thus supporting your blood counts.
2. If your ovaries aren't active, the thought is that they will absorb less chemo, making them more likely to turn back on and function after treatment is complete. I thought about it, and initially agreed. But over time it just did not sit well with me. I had spent the past three and a half years *supporting* my hormones and I was about to go through chemo—I just didn't want to do it.

Turns out, the painful recovery time was just what I needed; time to think. Because it took me so long to recover and because I was facing my first chemo infusion within a few weeks, that was enough to push me into listening to my instincts again. And my instincts said *not* to take that shot; I simply didn't want to stress my body out more than it already was. Also, the thought of hot flashes during chemo was not looking attractive. So I decided to support my body through treatment the best way I was able, and if my ovaries got damaged they got damaged. I knew I had 21 viable eggs to fall back on and decided if we ever want to use them we can, and if it didn't work, then in that case it's not God's plan.

This ended up being the right decision for me. Not only did I avoid hot flashes during treatment, I continued my cycle, and, not to get too personal, but after treatment was done my lady parts were more lubricated and my libido was back on track! Had I taken that shot, this recovery time would have been much longer and much more difficult.

This isn't to say that there aren't hormone challenges or imbalances that I will ultimately have to deal with due to treatment, and it's also not to say that this is the right choice for everyone. But it was the right choice for me.

The moral of this long, drawn-out story, is that your gut instinct is your friend. And when you have a gut feeling for or against something during this process, try to tune into that and listen. Sometimes your subconscious mind knows better than your conscious mind does.

We get really good at squishing that part of ourselves that tells us: "You can't do life alone". Or when it tells us to go to bed early, take a nap, eat a salad, do the hard thing, or force ourselves out of our comfort zone. This becomes dangerous when that still small voice is trying to speak up for itself and we refuse to listen by marrying the wrong man… ahem… I mean making a choice about our healthcare that really doesn't sit well with our deep self.

Keep a journal

When I got the diagnosis of Hodgkin lymphoma, my brain shut down and my ears closed up. You know how in movies when someone goes into shock the sound changes, dramatic music plays, and the person in front of them is talking away but the main character is in another world? Yeah. That happens in real life. Even if you do listen to something, you're probably going to forget it as your brain begins processing all the big important pieces of information. A journal can be an amazing tool to not only write down your questions and bring them into the office with you, but to keep track of dates, write down what tests or treatments are recommended, and generally document each part of the process while you are still in the office and can ask follow up questions.

It can also become therapeutic for you if you choose to use it as a tool to get all your thoughts and feelings onto the page whenever you are overwhelmed or want to remember a certain experience.

Find friends and resources to guide you and keep you positive

I would encourage you to reach out to friends and connections who can help you with this process of treatment and recovery and would be willing to support you regularly by text, phone call, or whatever works for you. That doesn't mean they are your therapist through the process, but having a support system is crucial!

I had a girlfriend who texted me regularly as I prepared to make my treatment decision and after I began treatment, and she would remind me of different questions I might want to ask the doctors. She would share her experiences with different medical testing and what to expect when I got there. This empowered me to be my own advocate, and helped me prepare for what I was about to experience.

If you don't have someone like that, you can join online support groups where you will find tons of resources! In the back of this book there are links to download my free guides: "10 questions to ask your oncologist", and "3 things you need to know when diagnosed with Hodgkin's". In addition to those resources I created a group on Facebook called "Healthy Through Hodgkin's" where I share information on healthy living, detoxing, information on integrative care and more.

There are other public Facebook groups for Hodgkin's patients that are more peer-to-peer led and you can either post a question you have about treatment, or search the group to see what others have shared and experienced. My only warning to you about those groups is this: while very helpful in many cases, they can also be a little scary. Many people talk about recurrence, nasty side effects, and they will share stories or pictures that make you think, "Will this happen to me?" I simply didn't want that in my newsfeed while I was going through this myself and so I generally avoided those groups during my treatment.

That's one of the main reasons I created "Healthy Through Hodgkin's" because I wanted there to be a platform that was focused on positive information that empowered the patient and would only put hopeful things in your newsfeed if you join. I really believe that maintaining a positive mentality is half the battle! You *must* believe that you will get well!

Don't be bullied

In the spirit of empowering women, one thing that grinds my gears is the fear surrounding cancer and the lack of encouragement and sometimes even lack of information from the doctor. Look, I had a great oncologist. I really like her. BUT. She's in this conventional medical world where she is legally limited in what she can say, recommend, and do. Heck, I had to practically drag it out of her that my clear PET scan meant that I was in remission.

You're probably not going to receive a lot of encouragement from your oncologist. They see so many cases, some good, some bad, some awful. They don't feel comfortable giving you false hope which means they often don't give you *much* hope.

You must maintain hope and inform yourself through the process. Read books, listen to podcasts, reach out to others in remission (way to go reading this book!) but whatever you do, know that you have options and what the doctor says or tells you may not be the whole (or only) story.

For example, with a few exceptions, there is no need to rush into treatment when you get a Hodgkin's diagnosis. Did you know that similar to an autoimmune disease, cancer begins developing in your body seven to ten years prior to getting symptoms or a diagnosis?

THAT TUMOR DID NOT JUST SHOW UP OVERNIGHT! I repeat. Whatever stage you find yourself in, this is not something that "just happened".

Already being immersed in the functional medicine world, I had a hunch that this lump had been in my neck way before I felt it. So I looked at my iPhone and searched old photos by dates and years, and sure enough... there were pictures from up to two years prior where I saw the lump in my neck. It was there, plain as day! God simply didn't allow me to see it until I was ready.

Whichever route you decide to go with for treatment, whether it be completely alternative and holistic, completely conventional, or in my case integrative, you must feel at peace with your decision. You must believe that it's the right decision for you. So take the time you need to gather the information that will help you feel most comfortable moving forward.

I know that everyone in your life will have an opinion. And when you take this time, those closest to you may even begin to freak out a little and push you towards whatever method they believe in and understand.

My decision-making process went something like this. I wanted to know what treatments there were, how effective they were for my specific cancer, and what testimonials I could find.

Here's the thing: I 100 per cent did find cases of women with Hodgkin's who lived with, or reversed their cancer by managing it strictly through diet and lifestyle. However, and this is part of what's tricky about the non-conventional world, much of this information is censored, and much is not supported (obviously) by big pharma, or large companies. This means that while alternative treatments and therapies exist, there aren't many studies you can find, and it's like looking for a needle in a haystack trying to find concrete evidence supported by strong statistics and recovery rates along with some solid testimonials for non-conventional treatments. When I found women that were managing their Hodgkin's through lifestyle it seemed excessively strict, and in one specific testimonial it seems like if she got a little lazy in her lifestyle her cancer would begin to grow again so she had to constantly be vigilant. I really didn't want to *live* with Hodgkin's the rest of my life.

On the other hand, I had solid statistics with conventional medicine showing that unlike many other cancers, Hodgkin's was a cancer that could not only be knocked out by chemotherapy, but the recurrence rate was also very low.

So I weighed my options. I could travel away from my family to live in an alternative care facility (there are many in the United States, some in Tijuana, Mexico, and others throughout the world... see the resources chapter), pay for everything out of pocket, and hope it worked. Or, I could go the conventional medicine route, knock it out in three months, support my body as much as I could through the process, and do everything I knew how to do to recover and get back to living my life.

I chose to do the latter. Whether you choose to move to a clinic or use chemotherapy it's OK. I only want you to know that there are options that fit within your lifestyle, belief system and budget that can align with your goals. And that's the biggest thing. Whatever treatment you choose, you must fully believe that it can help you.

In addition to chemotherapy my treatment plan included many supplements, emotional energy work, and spiritual growth. I'll talk more about these in the next chapters, but if you only take one thing away from this book, I want it to be this: You have within you the strength and the power to choose, and whatever decision you end up making is the right one for you. That intuition you are feeling leaning one way or the other—that's God trying to speak to you. We live in a culture where we are so busy, so distracted, so bombarded with schedules and technology that often it's difficult to hear that still small voice. So lean into that gut reaction. Listen to that intuition. Allow the Holy Spirit to speak loudly so that when you begin treatment you are in complete alignment with who you are and what you want. This can only assist you through the healing process.

3

―――

Treatment

POSSIBLY ONE OF the most difficult things to do, is just start treatment. I remember going to CTCA and feeling so out of place, sitting in a waiting room with actual sick people. "I don't belong here". "I'm not one of them". "I'm not sick like they are". I felt so healthy. So normal.

And then I walked into the chemo ward at my local hospital and it was almost revolting. Not the nurses, or the patients, but the concept. These patients looked so sick, unhappy, and unhealthy. Do I really want to be here? From January to May when I was hopping from doctor to doctor and hospital to hospital, I really grew to dislike being in that environment. But I had to get over it because this is what I chose to do. I had to face it and power through. So I started. And then so did treatment life.

OH. MY. WORD. The supplements. The nausea. The weird food aversions. Life changes a lot during treatment that is for sure. I will tell you straight up—I don't think there is any way you can get through treatment without feeling like total garbage at some point. But, I want to encourage you that you can support your body in a powerful way so that you do not feel as bad as you thought you would, you can recover quickly, and hopefully, even feel better at some points during treatment than you felt before! Yep, totally happened to me. There were actually weeks where I was like "Why do I feel so good?! This can't be normal". I think part of this may be because the more you remove the burden of stress (in this case the cancer itself) the better your body feels. It may also have to do with the extra oomph your body makes as it produces new, fresh blood after the counts have dropped so low. I may never know, but it certainly was a welcome reprieve!

My treatment schedule looked like this:

- Chemo every other Friday.
- The Saturday and Sunday after would be mostly sleeping, taking nausea meds and taking some walks but definitely a ton of Netflix. Like, whole seasons in one day... it was intense binging going on right there!
- The following Monday I would do my best to get off nausea meds (sometimes I needed a little longer) and get back to normal-ish life.
- The next Tuesday to Thursday I continued trying to get back to normal but would take it really easy if I needed to. I really tried not to schedule anything with other people until a full week after treatment.
- Somewhere in that week I would go to a clinic and get a Vitamin C IV.
- Friday after treatment to the Thursday before the next treatment: This was a full week to 10 days of feeling almost normal and in some rounds, feeling really great! The only round that I didn't get this wonderful recovery period was the second treatment.

Remember how I previously said listen to your gut instinct? There is a supplement called Biocidin that I use with my clients that is a magical antimicrobial, antiviral, antibiotic and is a great gut support supplement. It's herbal, gentle, and works on everything from sinus infections to major gut pathogens without killing all the beneficial gut bugs we need. Since I was working with my integrative oncologist and was taking supplements to protect my heart, lungs, muscles etc....from the chemo, I thought I would just drop Biocidin for now and just go with the cancer protocol. I mean... I'll do a lot to help my body but this was a *lot*! Let's keep it simple right?

I should have listened to my gut and never stopped taking it because after I received my port placement (the plastic device inserted into my chest with a catheter wrapping around and down into a vein where they would deliver the chemo) I had a really hard time healing fully. The incision just would not heal in one corner. Whether it was the suture knot itself or the material the stitch was made of, who knows... my body just didn't like it.

So after my immune system got knocked down after the second treatment, all the scary things started happening... my hair began falling out really quickly, my port infection got worse, and after spending a day lying in bed with stomach pains and a fever I ended up in the ER.

My white blood cell count was through the roof and I ended up spending the night in the hospital getting an antibiotic delivered by IV every six hours. Let me share something about sleeping in a hospital; it is literally the *worst* experience. I value my sleep. Over a lot of things. I *love* sleep. I guard my sleep.

I used to be a total night owl and think sleeping in was ok until I discovered I was violating my natural circadian rhythm and how unhealthy that actually was for me... long story short... I now really value sleep. And the hospital won't let you get any. At all.

This approach really confuses me because sleep is where our cells and muscles regenerate and where our brain and body detoxifies the best... don't sick people need the most restful sleep possible?

I mean, I get coming in to check on a patient to make sure they are breathing and their vitals are normal on the little beeping machine... But do you really have to wake me up every one or two hours to get my blood pressure, stick me with another shot, or ask me questions? I mean...

Needless to say, the next day I was feeling better (thanks antibiotics!) so I asked if I could take a pill form of the antibiotics and go home. The doctor agreed and sent me home with two insanely strong antibiotics.

Hold up! Kylene, you are a functional health coach! You work on healing guts and avoiding antibiotics and you said *yes* to *two* antibiotics? Well, yes... sort of... jeez, let me get back to the story!

I believe there is a time and place for conventional medicine. Even ones that can be toxic or harmful on some level, depending on the circumstance. When you are getting chemotherapy, one of the most toxic treatments you can possibly get on your body and one of the *most* damaging to your immune system, infections are nothing to sniff at. So yes, I took the antibiotics.

However, I didn't feel like I needed both of them and I could tell that it was overkill. I wasn't feeling that great taking two so I called my oncologist and asked if it was ok to drop the one I thought was making me feel bad. She agreed and I continued the 10 days on the single antibiotic.

Remember that little herbal tincture I was telling you about? Well once I got off of the RX antibiotic, you better believe that I got right back onto that tincture and I never had any other problems!

This is where I pause and reiterate that it's important to work with your doctor or practitioner for these things. Don't go randomly taking stuff you've never used before. I had used Biocidin regularly, knew how amazing it was and had already talked to my integrative oncologist about including it.

I was also taking a probiotic daily throughout treatment, and once I took the antibiotics I added another one with different strains to help recover my precious microbiome. This was in addition to other supplements in my protocol that were designed to help soothe and heal my gut lining.

Because of this interruption in my normal recover, then feel pretty good, and then go back to treatment schedule, I didn't really get the mental and physical recovery time during that second round which was hard. Physically, you want to be as strong as you can going into your next chemo because mentally you want to feel like you can take another hit. This was really the only round I didn't feel like I got that. I did hear later from several people that the second round is typically the hardest and that was true for me too. So if that happens to you, keep your spirits up, the worst is most likely behind you!

Everyone's journey will be different. Some people end up in the hospital several times, and others will never have a blip in treatment. Your health history, your immune system, your lifestyle is unique, so don't let it discourage you either way.

My encouragement however, is that there are so many things we can do to strengthen our bodies and minds through this otherwise scary process. You can achieve the best health possible during and after treatment regardless of where you're coming from.

Are you reading this before treatment? Great! Take some time to assemble your team (next chapter!). Are you reading this during treatment? Jump to the resource chapter or read the rest of this book to incorporate what you're able to, when you're able to. Any step forward is a step in the right direction.

Your number one priority right now is your health. And you're the only one that can take charge of that.

4

Assemble your team

EVERY DOCTOR NEEDS a doctor, every coach needs a coach, and every athlete needs a trainer. If the President of the United States needs advisors then why, when facing the biggest challenge in our lives, would we be any different?

I knew as soon as I heard the diagnosis that I needed a team. I already knew that my diet was important, my mindset was critical, and my emotional health was key. But I also knew that I needed others to support and guide me through this.

I'm going to be blatantly honest with you and say my husband and I threw a *lot* of money at this. But you don't have to. You can hire the best coaches in the world and create your team of rock stars, or you can utilize free resources like books and podcasts (see the resource chapter) and design your own plan.

Your team includes anyone in your corner: spouse, friends, family, oncologist, personal trainer, emotional energy healer, pastor, author, health coach etc.... your team might look completely different than my team but I'll share with you what I did and why. Please take from it what *you* need.

The first person I got on board was the integrative oncologist Dr. Heather Paulson. I liked her because she came highly recommended and could work with me throughout the treatment based on what I needed whether that be getting on the phone after each treatment (or every other) or shooting her an email in between. I also felt drawn to her because her husband had beaten Hodgkin's and she had been with him through that experience so she knew first-hand what was going on. If you feel there is no one in your area that offers this, take heart! We met long-distance by phone or video chat!

Next was the oncologist—obviously. But this is really important. Don't think just because you got assigned an oncologist that you can't find another one. When my ENT specialist said he was referring me, I flat out said to him on the phone: "Hey, I just want to say, I'll be utilizing nutrition through this process so I need someone who will support that." He replied, "Oh you will love Dr. N. She is a vegan, and I really think you will like her". So I totally lucked out! My oncologist saw my supplement list and I told her I was working with a naturopath specializing in oncology and as long as I communicated with her what I was doing she was fine with it. Find a doctor like that. One that will support *you* in the way *you* want to be supported.

I went to a clinic periodically to get intravenous Meyers Cocktails (a blend of magnesium, B vitamins and vitamin C) before my cancer diagnosis, so I asked if I could switch to Vitamin C only. Please note: I approved this through my integrative oncologist and I chose to have these between chemo treatments. While the extra vitamins in the Meyers Cocktail are wonderful, Vitamin C IV treatments are given at a much higher dose than you would get from a Meyers blend. This therapy has been shown to not only assist the chemotherapy in fighting the cancer, but also in mitigating some of the negative effects as well.

Next, I worked with someone who practiced emotional code therapy and some other bioenergetics work. I had heard from several in the functional medicine and alternative health world that emotions are often connected to cancer. For example, Fran Drescher (yes the Nanny!) attributes the development of her uterine cancer to being raped at gunpoint when she was younger. The resulting trapped trauma so to speak, may be what weakened

> ### *Important note*
>
> While rare, there is a condition where vitamin C IVs can actually kill you. It's a rare deficiency that you need to have tested and it's called G6PD. If you already have a genetic test like 23andme it's easy to check! If not, you can request a blood test from your oncologist.

that area of her body and triggered the development of cancer. These things can be difficult to prove but if you are someone who has experienced a lot of stress or trauma it's worth considering.

I'll discuss the emotional and physical connection more later, but in my mind if there was some emotion that I was holding onto, or some trauma that needed to be healed in order for my body to heal, I wanted to make sure that I pursued every path open to me.

Finally, I hired a detox specialist. Unfortunately, because of the timing of the fertility treatments and then how quickly the chemo started I wasn't able to begin utilizing her until after treatment which in the end, was perfect timing! (God always knows).

My family was another incredible asset in my team. My husband is ultra-supportive in every aspect of my life. Facing this challenge down was no exception, and he was there to wait on me hand and foot every weekend after treatment.

My Dad came to every single chemo infusion. In addition, I had at least one friend at every infusion as well. My sisters came (and one even travelled) to come to some of my treatments.

My Mom made me dinner every Friday and Saturday during the week of treatment.

My church prayed earnestly for me, and so did my sister and brother-in-law's church, as well as Christians and friends around the country.

I received messages, cards, DMs and gifts from those on Facebook who have followed me or known me for a long time.

I received a blanket from an employee that works for my husband.

I received gift baskets from women at my church.

My girlfriend set up a meal train and people showed up out of the blue to bring delicious and healthy meals to my door the days following treatment.

I'm not saying this as someone who is an 'influencer' or famous because... I'm not. On any level. In fact, the support blew me out of the water. I'm a total nobody. And yet so many cared.

And so many care for you. This will be, in the midst of the fire, a beautiful time to say "yes" to accepting help. Recognizing those around you who really love and care for you. To even reach out and *ask* for help which may be hard, but it is important. Let those people serve you. Allow yourself to relax. Utilize the resources and people in your life that are available to you and never feel selfish. This, of all the times in your life, is a time to prioritize rest, healing, stress relief, and relaxation.

There are online communities you can reach out to for encouragement and support. There are websites, blogs and Facebook groups like I mentioned previously.

A quick note on finding your tribe. As difficult as cancer is, the love and support we receive can be addictive, especially if it's support that we have always craved but never received. If this is you, don't allow yourself to fall into "victim" mode where you subconsciously sabotage your ability to heal because you are enjoying the attention too much.

That might sound shocking, harsh, or even mean. But it's a real phenomenon and in her book *Why People Don't Heal* Caroline Myss coined it "woundology".

Different personalities are more or less susceptible to this–even me! As an Enneagram 3 (a personality type based on the Enneagram system) I love affirmation and attention. I mean, I'm a performer and former opera singer after all, and my love language is verbal affirmation and gift receiving!

But if you catch yourself falling into this trap, remind yourself that you would rather be healthy no matter what! You must remember who you are throughout this process. **This disease does not define you**. It's simply a door you must walk through.

If you're more of an introvert, or don't find that you have a wave of support wrapped around you, make sure that you reach out. Your church, friends, or even online support groups are available to help. lls.org provides cancer buddies if you would like to talk with someone that is around your age and has previously been through the same cancer.

In the end you may find, as I did, that you walk away from this with an amazing community of love and support that you never realized existed.

5

Hodgkin's does not define you

I HAD MORE time than most to mentally prepare for this process. One thing I knew right away was that I did not want this disease to become so all-encompassing that it began to define who I was. I wasn't going to let it beat me mentally *or* physically.

Even with that determination I found myself slipping into that all too easy mindset... my life, my daily patterns, my thoughts... *everything* was revolving around treatment or recovery. I was slowly losing who I was as I began to live the "cancer life".

It's really hard not to. The day my hair began falling out was incredibly traumatic. It was immediately after the second dose of chemotherapy and I remember stepping out of the shower, and looking down to see hair all over my chest and arms. I had hoped that this wouldn't happen until much later. I texted my husband, who rushed home and held me as I cried and cried. I had him buzz my head that night because I didn't want to experience the slow agony of watching this happen day after day after day. I sat there with a red, puffy face as my husband carefully removed the last bit of my femininity, and what I felt, was part of my identity.

I had been growing my hair longer for years, before cutting it into a pixie length when I got diagnosed. I felt weird, and unfeminine then, and when I shaved it off that just accentuated the awkward and insecure feelings I had. None of this is easy. What is easy, however, is to become consumed by the dozens of emotions you feel every single day of this process.

About halfway through treatments, this cancer mindset really started to annoy me. I wasn't feeling like myself anymore. Maybe it hit me because I had my 33rd birthday and six-year marriage anniversary almost right at the halfway mark of treatment, or maybe I just got tired of being poopy. Either way, I decide to make a change.

The first thing I did was find something that made me happy. Singing makes me happy. So I downloaded a karaoke app (SMULE I'm on there as-Kylene Terhune if anyone wants to connect!) and started recording songs. It immediately began working to get me out of my funk!

Singing speaks to my soul. It hits me on a deeper level and resonates in my whole being. So when I started singing again, even alone in my home to an app on my phone, I began to feel better.

I also decided that while I still needed to be careful, I couldn't just avoid people and be a hermit throughout this process. Whether that meant I fist bumped in public to avoid hugging and shaking hands, stayed away from big crowds, and took showers when I got home, fine. But darn it, I was going to get together with other humans.

And finally, my neighbor recommended a local Pilates class and I incorporated movement back into my life. Movement and exercise was always a huge part of my life (I was a part-time personal trainer up until my diagnosis), yet for most of the year I hadn't done much as we waded through diagnosis, staging, testing and treatment. I began going to a Pilates class a couple of times a week, and this, in addition to my daily walking, was the perfect amount of gentle movement for where I was physically at that time.

From the beginning of treatment I made sure to get outside and walk every single day. Some days I would be able to get out several times with my husband and our dog Cocoa, or sometimes it would just be me and Cocoa, but it was my goal to at least get out of bed and take a short walk no matter what.

This was a major slow down from my normal amount of activity, so adding in Pilates classes really helped me mentally feel better!

If you are beginning to feel the slump, I would encourage you to really dig into what makes you happy. What did you really enjoy before treatment? And how can you incorporate it in a safe way again?

For some of you it may be gardening to get your hands back in the dirt. For others it might be music, or art, or going out for coffee with a friend. Whatever it is, try to incorporate more joy back into your day. Be intentional about it. Being around other people can be tremendously helpful when it's the *right* people. Make sure you choose your companions and outings wisely, and make sure you continue to *live* your life through this journey. You are still you. Fill your cup with things that make you feel like yourself.

Think future thoughts

People don't live long without hope. Plain and simple. You can have the sickest person in the world defy all diagnoses by living well beyond the predicted amount of time that their body should hold out, simply because they have a life purpose and hope.

My Grandmother transitioned from earth to heaven a few years ago and while her body began shutting down, she lay silent and still for days in the bed unable to communicate, move or speak. She held on however, until the last of her children had had a chance to say goodbye, and then she slipped peacefully away.

There is so much that we can't comprehend about the power of the mind, holding on to hope and living into your purpose. Those things are crucial through a healing journey.

I mentioned that about halfway through treatment it was my birthdaversary week, and while I scheduled my treatments to leave that weekend free, I was so sad that I wouldn't be able to take my normal vacation with Patrick to celebrate. I look forward to that trip every year because we choose something new and fun to do and we get a whole week together, just us. I start craving it when we haven't traveled recently enough, and I realized that the trip would be delayed this year.

But it gave me something to look forward to when treatment was completed! We regularly talked about where we wanted to take our birthdaversary-remission-celebration trip! And yes, long silly titles make everything *way* more fun.

We talked about Italy and it provided fun research and a beautiful mental escape for me to think about. Ultimately, we decided to go to Quebec and enjoy some beautiful time in an old monastery-turned-wellness center, followed by a stay in a historical hotel built in the 1600s.

Throughout the treatment year we were also building our dream house, and so I had home meetings that I would schedule on my better weeks, and I could think about cabinets and flooring and fun things like that.

Now, I'm not saying to go build your dream house in the middle of chemotherapy! But beyond whatever activities bring you joy that you can incorporate today, what are some events or life moments that you look forward to when you're healthy?

It could be as simple as focusing on being healthy for a child's birthday party, or celebrating Christmas with your family knowing that you won't have any more treatments. Maybe it *is* a fancy vacation to celebrate your victory, or maybe it's taking some classes, or opening your own business.

This process will be one of many spiritual revelations if you are open to it. You will find yourself contemplating your purpose, your message, your ministry, your calling... Find what lights you up and think on it often.

Visualization has been used for ages as a tool to calm, to heal, and to focus the mind. Beyond simply making you think happy thoughts, this hopeful thinking can become a critical asset to your healing journey.

6

Optimizing Nutrition

LET'S TALK ABOUT some practical, physical, delicious and easy ways you can support your body during and after treatment!

Google. Isn't there so much fun information out there about what to eat during chemo? Eat meat, no don't eat meat. Eat butter, no don't eat butter, it will kill you. Eat only vegetables, no don't eat vegetables...

Before we dive into the nuances that chemotherapy brings to the table, let's talk about my overall nutrition perspective. I teach #YOUtrition. That's right, #YOUtrition because there is no one diet that works for every single human being. Add on top of it a treatment like chemo-therapy and you have a lot to think about, from dealing with nausea, to water tasting terrible, to new cravings to deal with.

While I don't believe there is one right diet for everyone, I do believe there are some guidelines that *do* work for everyone.

Let's begin with the idea that food is information. It gets broken down in your body and communicates different things. Carbohydrates get broken down and then get used as energy or stored in the liver as glucose (energy) for later. Fat helps cushion your organs, create hor-mones, make healthy cell structures, and fat feeds your brain. Protein helps maintain muscle mass, repair tissues, and helps lots of important chemical reactions happen correctly in the body.

Let's build on that concept and add that a calorie is not just a calorie. Vitamins, minerals and enzymes work most efficiently when complete in their natural form. This is because they come neatly packaged up with other vitamins, minerals and enzymes that work together in synergy to create specific processes in the body, to cancel each other out, or to help your body assimilate them most efficiently. So yes, there is a huge difference between a Pop Tart with 200 calories, 3g of protein, 36g of carbohydrate and 1.5g of fat, and a baked sweet potato with grass-fed butter and broccoli with the same "calories" and macro content.

One of those options comes loaded with inflammatory ingredients, sugar, and lack of nutrients. The other comes with anti-inflammatory ingredients, zero added sugar, and tons of nutrients. All wrapped up in a perfect package to be delivered efficiently into your body in a healthy way.

Are you beginning to vibe with me on how important these day-to-day choices are, especially when facing something as toxic and inflammatory as chemotherapy?

When your body is under stress, any stress really, but for our purposes, cancerous stress, the last thing we want to do is add more inflammation, more stress, more effort, more things for it to think about. Alternatively, what we *want* to do is give it every benefit, tool, resource, vitamin and mineral we possibly can so that while it's working hard it can focus on what it needs to, and pull from the bucket of resources we offer.

Another way to visualize this is to think of the foods we eat as building blocks for our cells, which in turn are the building blocks for our whole body. When our goal is to build a strong, healthy, resilient and disease free body, we had better be using reinforced concrete blocks instead of foam bricks! The trouble is, our body is incredibly intelligent and resourceful. For awhile, it can use the foam bricks to create stability, and it will "cheat" so to speak to get what it needs. Ultimately however, the foam bricks fail, leaving holes in the wall and eventually those walls fall down. Just because we don't have a heart attack the moment we eat a sleeve of Oreos, doesn't mean they aren't causing harm.

Begin to look at the food on your plate and ask the questions: Is this food feeding, fueling, and strengthening my cells? Is it nutrient dense? Or nutrient void?

To get a detailed breakdown of foods and nutrients that can be helpful during cancer, I highly recommend the book *Beating Cancer with Nutrition* by Patrick Quillin.

For now, let's talk about the big, overarching principles that I discuss with my clients on a regular basis. These are all recommendations made by me. I am not a nutritionist or dietitian, but have utilized these principles with myself, my clients and my family for years with only positive results. Again, the goal is to remove as many stressors as we can, while providing the body with as many nutrients as possible.

If you're reading this in the middle of treatment then making these changes may seem overwhelming in your already exhausted state. Do what you can when you can. Perhaps this is information that you absorb now and implement later. Or perhaps you can take one tidbit now and go on from there. Do what works for you.

Gluten-free

The single food (it's a protein actually) that I am hard-core about with my clients, is gluten. It's the only food that I tell every human to avoid like the plague. Seriously. I've never really met anyone that doesn't feel better OFF of it except one or two people and I actually believe there were some other nutrient deficiencies and imbalances happening there.

Because foods affect everyone differently, everyone experiences different benefits from eliminating wheat/gluten from their diet. These can include but are not limited to:

- Weight loss (especially in the belly)
- More energy
- Clearer skin
- More balanced moods
- Less inflammation
- Clearer thinking (less brain fog)
- Better bowel movements

This isn't a science book *or* a nutrition book, so I won't get super deep (if you'd like more in-depth information, see the resources section) but there are a few reasons I am so committed to this one:

1. Wheat has several proteins (including gluten) that cause negative reactions in us. Gluten specifically raises the level of a protein called zonulin which increases the permeability of the gut which can lead to inflammation. The *last* thing you need during chemo is extra inflammation. What you *need* is foods that heal and soothe the gut! Since chemo damages your fast dividing cells it also damages your intestinal lining. Eating foods like gluten pile onto this effect instead of helping it recover more quickly.
2. Wheat is a heavily glyphosate (pesticide) sprayed crop. Tiny microscopic particles of glyphosate have been shown to negatively impact your good gut bugs. In addition, glyphosate is now being linked to the development of cancer. We want to eliminate this stressor and protect our gut bugs!

3. Over time, wheat has been hybridized, and the gluten protein has more than doubled. Add that to the exponential increase of processed foods, almost all of which include wheat, and your exposure has skyrocketed over the years! No wonder all these gluten sensitivities are popping up.

Gluten is probably the #1 food sensitivity that people see the most benefit in eliminating. The best part is, they usually see it quickly and dramatically too!

Processed foods

Now I know that this can be hard when we are busy, tired, or stressed from treatment. But I'm not eliminating *all* premade and packaged foods here. I'm simply eliminating processed foods that have artificial ingredients, added sugars or gluten in them.

A simple read of the label should answer this question: "Could I technically make this at home?" If you can recognize all the ingredients and they are real foods then the answer is yes. Yay!

Brands like Simple Mills are excellent at creating pancakes, muffins, crackers and breads with five ingredients or less, all of which you could technically buy yourself. Get familiar with your grocery store and what brands they carry that might be similar!

Cutting out processed foods does eliminate most fast food restaurants since their ingredients are low quality, and gluten hides in the most random places (hello Taco Bell menu). The oils used are often inflammatory oils such as canola or safflower oil.

I like to rate fast food restaurants on different levels as real life means we sometimes want or need something fast. Below is how I would score some of the most popular options:

NEVER:

> McDonalds
> Taco Bell
> Arby's

IN A PINCH:

> Wendy's
> Burger King
> 5 Guys

OFTEN

> Chipotle
> Whole Foods salad bar

I would encourage you to do your own research! Look up what different restaurant ingredients are and go from there!

Increase produce and real food intake

Regardless of where you are in life, this is the biggie. This is the main priority. Real food should always make up most of your diet. And by real food I mean, can it pass this simple question test: "Was it made in a factory? Or was it made by the earth?"

Vegetables, roots and tubers should be the foundation of every meal! Fruits, veggies, beans, legumes and nuts are on the list, as well as healthy fats like avocado, coconut and grass-fed butter. Wild-caught fish, grass-fed meat etc..... That's a real food diet!

If this is all new for you, you won't be able to incorporate it all at once in the middle of treatment, but set some goals and take some steps.

Continue to research and find blogs and recipes to use as you heal, and when you're in remission so you can begin to support your body a little more each day.

Special note on produce

When your blood counts are low and your immune system is compromised, it's a little more risky to eat raw fruits and veggies due to the increased risk of bacterial exposure. Washing does not always remove the threat, so steam or cook your veggies and choose fruits with a thick skin that you don't eat like melons, and then discard the skin. I recommend avoiding berries during this time. Always check with your doctor if you have concerns about this.

Love your liver

Your liver is so amazing. Can you just stop for a moment and thank your liver for everything that it does for you on a daily basis? It's this incredible detoxifier for our bodies and it's so easy to become unaware of what we are burdening it with!

One day, when my blood counts were low, and a liver enzyme was a little high, my nurse called to let me know and she said, "So don't be drinking alcohol this week." I remember thinking: "Who drinks alcohol during chemo?" But the fact that she felt the need to throw that out there says that someone, somewhere, drinks through treatment.

So, let me give you some tough love here my friend. Don't be the person who drinks during chemo. Regardless of your bloodwork numbers! Love. That. Liver.

Everything you do during and after treatment should be about loving your liver and giving your cells the nutrients they need to heal quickly, and to attack the bad guys. Sorry to say this, but alcohol, sugar, additives and processed foods do *not* do that. They just stress your liver and kidneys and give your body *more* to detoxify.

That doesn't mean you can't have a little treat here and there. There was a whole day after treatment one time that all I wanted was ice cream bars. Did they have sugar? Yes they did. But I chose gluten-free and dairy-free options to make the best choice possible, while listening to my body, and balancing my diet as soon as I could after that. Phew! Now that *that* elephant is out of the room...

Always listen to your body: You may find you have super-weird cravings and it's possible your body needs a nutrient so it's asking for it through these little signals. Or maybe your mouth is sore after treatment and cold ice cream is all that feels good. It's ok to live a little. I just want every choice you make to be a conscious choice.

Your liver has two phases of detoxification. The first is where it uses enzymes to make toxins, well, not toxic anymore. Ironically, the by-products of that process can also be unhealthy for your body, so you have a second phase of detoxification where your liver then breaks everything down that's toxic or marked for excretion. This makes it harmless to your body and water-soluble so it can be removed efficiently. Pretty cool huh?

Both phases require lots and lots of nutrients including B vitamins, glutathione, antioxidants, Vitamins C and E and amino acids.

To make it easy you can think about it this way: Phase one really needs fruits and vegetables and phase two needs proteins!

Let's talk about a few foods you could incorporate to support your liver and love it more if you do have a raised enzyme level at any point. (P.S. these foods would be great to have always!)

Onions
Broccoli
Cauliflower
Asparagus
Berries
Leafy greens
Grass-fed red meat, pasture-raised poultry and eggs, wild-caught fish
Organic, vegan protein shakes (easy on the digestion)

Remember, during treatment fruits and vegetables should probably be cooked! If you really enjoy soft fruits or berries, try making a compote! This is easily done by heating the berries on low heat until they get soft enough to mush up. You can sweeten with a little honey, but if they are really ripe you may not need to!

Coffee

Coffee deserves a special note because it's so popular and because cancer, and treatment, makes you really tired. While it may be tempting to rely more and more on a caffeinated beverage, that only adds more stress to your body. Coffee (or any caffeine) stimulates your adrenal glands to release more cortisol which gives you that energy bump. But our adrenal glands are very sensitive to stress, and caffeine is a stressor. Since this is a stressor we *can* control, I recommend limiting your coffee to one cup of black coffee before noon.

If you'd like to utilize whatever cortisol you are producing in the morning and get the most out of your coffee for the day, then simply wait to drink it after you've been awake for one hour.

I always recommend stopping at noon because caffeine has a long circulating half-life, which means that it continues to break down in your body and circulate in lesser and lesser amounts until it's gone. For a few fast metabolizers, this may happen fairly quickly, but if you are a slow metabolizer (or under stress) then the half-life can last upwards of eight hours, ultimately disturbing your sleep if it's in your body too late.

You can find what works for you, but I found myself avoiding coffee for a few days after treatment, and then drinking it again three to four days later. Taking into consideration that the days following treatment are when you need the most rest, you don't want to add any potential stress to your liver or stop yourself from sleeping!

Everyone's recovery pattern is different however, so once you've been through a few rounds of treatment, you'll recognize the patterns and be able to adjust accordingly.

I should probably mention sodas and teas as well! Soda would fall within the avoid-all-processed-foods recommendation previously. Even diet sodas contain high amounts of fake ingredients and sweeteners that are linked to cancer. They also contain phosphoric acid which has been linked to poor bone health! Best to avoid soda altogether whether in or out of treatment. Zevia is a chemical and sugar free brand of soda that tastes great if you are looking for a soda swap!

Tea can be very healing and have many different and beneficial uses depending on the herb used to make it. Green tea is often associated with cancer prevention and treatment because of EGCG which is a potent antioxidant. Since green tea is naturally caffeinated, I would recommend drinking it before noon for the same reasons as coffee.

Eating around treatment

Oh boy! The food aversions you may have read or heard about, are REAL. But surprisingly, for me, so were the cravings! I am someone that likes to be prepared so I bought a cookbook about eating for cancer, and I was like *yes*! I'm going to make these recipes, it tells me what foods to eat the week after treatment to get extra nourishment, I'm gonna DO THIS!

And then I had my first treatment and discovered that what you eat during treatment will probably be out for a good long while after... You have a good chance of getting a negative food association with that food and your body won't want it. Don't worry, as you heal and your tummy gets back to normal you'll get your broader appetite back!

Here are some tips that I found helpful around treatment:

Water is so important!

Hydrate hydrate hydrate! Start the day before treatment, and drink as much as you can on the day *of* treatment. After that, water began to be difficult for me because it can taste funny. Because of all the chemicals and toxins from chemo some people describe the taste after treatment as metallic. Some also experience mouth sores which can also impact taste and ability to eat. We tried *everything*. We flavored water every which way and eventually I just had to force myself to get it down. Dehydration makes *everything* worse and while you can go in for a hydration IV which is incredibly helpful, it's much easier and cheaper to drink water – so don't skimp on that water! Do whatever it takes for the first two or three days after treatment to force it down until you can drink normally and it tastes ok again.

Hydration is extra important after chemo. Treatment and nausea medications can dehydrate you, and you want to stay ahead of the curve to avoid stronger side-effects as well as constipation and headaches.

Snacks during treatment

I highly recommend packing snacks for your chemotherapy infusions. I had a friend that only drank water during her treatment and I admire her. I have no idea how she did it because, personally, I had to eat like a pig during treatment to avoid feeling really nauseous. I would err on the safe side and pack some snacks just in case. On that note, try to pack foods you don't normally eat or that you won't eat the next few days since you may notice an aversion to them during that time.

There have been studies that show that fasting the day prior to treatment and then through treatment may assist the chemotherapy in doing its job and being even more effective.

There was *no way* my body could have handled it on an empty stomach, so while this may work for some, I would recommend packing those snacks. For me I would usually get to the hospital around 8-9am to see the doctor, and start treatment by 10-10:30am. They don't order the chemo drugs until your blood work comes back ok so there is some down time before receiving the infusion. If all goes well, the actual treatment takes another 3-4 hours.

Be flexible

In the beginning we tried to stock the pantry with foods we thought I might crave or need after treatment, but because of aversions and cravings (that seemed to change every dang time!) we eventually chilled out on that because I told my husband: "I'm just going to have to tell you what I want, when I want it, I'm sorry". I didn't want him going out and buying six boxes of grain-free crackers only to have me not want to eat them.

Do prepare a few things just in case. I found that plain food is what really did it for me. Plain meat, veggies with butter, maybe some gluten-free toast or nut butter with raisins... watermelon was a really big one for me. Oh the sweet, cool hydration of watermelon. But overall, nothing too fancy or seasoned. Simple seemed to work much better for me.

Balance your diet as soon as you can

Once the treatment aversions and cravings calm down, try to get back into your normal routine of a balanced diet. Getting back to this as quickly as possible and including your veggies can help with keeping your gut on track.

If you are able, I would incorporate foods like bone broth and sauerkraut. Bone broth is extremely nutritious and is soothing for your gut which gets a big hit during treatment. It's also a rich source of minerals and collagen.

A note on spices

For me, personally, because of the damage done to the epithelial lining in my throat, there were rounds where I was more sensitive to spices. This meant avoiding anything spicy was important, otherwise I would get a cold, burning sensation all down my throat. Not fun! Stick with salt unless you know you can tolerate spices.

If you do experience irritation after eating something spicy, drinking organic, whole leaf aloe juice may provide some relief.

Sauerkraut is a food-based probiotic which means it will get all the way through your system successfully. Each jar has slightly different strains and can help you stay balanced during treatment. Because it is a raw food you may want to ask your doctor if they are ok with you adding it into your diet.

Eating before you begin chemotherapy

Before treatment, is a good time to go nutrient crazy! Anytime we have the opportunity to build up our strength, fill our nutrient stores, and give our body some backup, we should take it!

Prioritize salads, green smoothies, green juices (avoid super sugary ones with tons of fruit!), all the vegetables, as much organic as possible (see the EWG clean 15 and dirty dozen to prioritize which produce is most important to buy organic). Just Google the Gerson Diet or The Green Smoothie Girl and you'll get tons of ideas!

Here's my favorite green juice (I promise it's yummy!):

- 1 organic honey crisp apple
- 2-3 kale stalks
- 2-3 organic celery stalks
- Nub of fresh ginger
- 1 organic lemon

Be careful as the ginger can be zippy!

Just push through a juicer, adding as much ginger as you like, to taste.

You can mix and match with juices as much as you want! Beet is really wonderful for your blood and acts as a good detoxifier. Apples are a great fruit to sweeten a smoothie without getting too sugary or over the top. You can add any leafy greens, carrots, or completely start from scratch! Juicing is a great way to get rid of extra produce at the end of the week before it goes bad as well.

Just make sure you thoroughly rinse everything before juicing it since it is a raw product.

Easy produce wash

Use this solution to wash your vegetables and fruits before eating raw or using them in a juice or smoothie.

- Water to cover produce
- ¼ cup white vinegar or apple cider vinegar
- 1 tbsp baking soda

Cover your produce in this mix and soak for 15 minutes. Rinse off and dry.

Some produce does soak up the water and gets a little soggy if you don't use it right away. I've noticed this with root veggies in particular. So just pay attention to which produce you use and decide whether or not you want to clean all your produce at once or do this just before you eat it.

You'll discover what flavors and combinations you really enjoy, and before you know it, you'll be craving your morning juice!

Eating in remission

Once you're in remission it's time to boost that immune system and support your liver! You can support your body's detox pathways in a natural and gentle way.

As you heal you may still consider cooking some of your veggies so not all the produce you have is raw (raw veggies are harder on digestion), but begin incorporating juices and salads back into your diet. Notice how your digestion changes and how your stomach feels when you do this. You may need to incorporate digestive enzymes or wait a little longer to eat raw veggies, based on how you feel. Do you get super gassy after a salad? You may want to slow down on the raw roughage for now.

You can focus on including great natural detoxifiers like broccoli sprouts, sauerkraut and beets and overall just try to get as much variety as possible. Don't just rotate between the old favorites peas, broccoli and green beans (I get it, we've all been there)... but instead try for as many different veggies as you can.

This is really an opportunity to try new things, experience new flavors, and embrace your new role as primary caregiver of your body. Every bite you put in your mouth can help boost your immune system or stress it out. So bring in those colors, fruits, nuts, seeds and beans and look at this as an adventure. I would even recommend standing in the produce section each week and looking for a new plant to try! Just Google how to cook it when you get home.

My favorite salad recipe

- Handful of organic mixed greens
- Handful of organic broccoli sprouts
- 1 or 2 organic veggies like tomatoes, mushrooms, carrots or cucumbers chopped
- 1-2 TBSOrganic red onion chopped
- 1-2 TBS Nutritional yeast (great source of B12 and it has a great "cheese" flavor!)
- Paleo ranch dressing (homemade is great, but Primal Kitchen also has a great grocery store option)

There are as many salad combination options as there are stars in the sky, so get creative (we can all get stuck with the same old favorites). Your salad base doesn't even have to be leafy greens! It could be a bowl of broccoli mixed with other veggies sprinkled with sesame seeds and dressed with coconut aminos (a great soy sauce alternative).

Just play. Enjoy your food. Thank God for the nutrition it will bring you and visualize the healing that occurs with every bite. Get out of the false mentality that "healthy" tastes bad and instead step into this rainbow-colored sparkle world that is fresh, beautiful produce. It is all designed to fuel your body in a way that heals your cells, fights cancer, boost energy, and helps you have beautiful hair, skin and nails!

Eating to support your gut

Ugh. One of the most common and annoying side effects of going through chemotherapy is the total devastation of your gut... and usually constipation at one point or another. Let's get into why your gut is hit so hard during treatment.

There is a lining of cells that covers your throat, nasal passages, stomach and small intestine. It's a mucosal layer, a layer of epithelial cells all lined up in a row. These cells are connected by what are called "tight junctions". These are fast-dividing cells just like your hair cells and cancer cells... this means that chemo targets them without discrimination, which is why we lose our hair, experience sensitivity to spices, feel weird in the sinuses, get headaches, and have tummy troubles during treatment.

The tight junctions are semi-permeable. That means that they open and close like those boat bridges that raise up and allow boats to pass at certain times. We want this cell lining to be semi-permeable because certain nutrients need to get into our blood stream through digestion. But we want it to be a highly controlled process. Not one that is accidental and caused by inflammation and damage to the cells.

Since the cells are most likely damaged during chemotherapy, that's another motivator to avoid highly processed, inflammatory foods during treatment since those foods can also irritate the gut and hinder the cell repair and healing process.

Because the epithelial cells are fast replicators, they die off and replace each other quickly too; every three to seven days you have a new gut lining. As long as it isn't over-burdened that is. The problem comes in when it gets damaged at a faster rate than it can recover. My goal was to support my gut lining to heal as quickly as it could in-between treatments. I incorporated several things to manage this process which I mention below.

For healing and support

20-30g/day of L Glutamine. L Glutamine is like repair fuel for those epithelial cells. It helps them repair and boy did I want to help them.

For soothing

One of the L Glutamine supplements I used contained 5g of L Glutamine in addition to herbs like marshmallow root, aloe and slippery elm to soothe the damaged tissues. This can also be helpful for acid reflux and spice sensitivity.

One treatment where I was particularly sensitive I added about 4oz of real aloe juice as well, for its soothing properties.

For better digestion and poop

Hydration is obviously important, but the reasons you get constipated during treatment are a little more complicated. Even a few days on your anti-nausea meds can do you in. Instead of taking something harsh to the stomach lining like Miralax or X-Lax, I chose to utilize Senokot which uses senna, an herb, to keep me regular during that time. I personally only needed it a few times, usually around the nausea meds, to stay on track. I would encourage you to find what works for you and be proactive. It may work really well to use something like this the night of treatment and then for the next few days as your adjust back to your normal diet, recover from the treatment, get hydrated, and wean off the nausea meds.

The old remedies are tried and true! Eating three to six dried prunes can really assist as well. This is something you could even snack on daily without worrying if it will be "too harsh" on your system.

I took a spore-based probiotic almost every night and that, in addition to eating probiotic rich foods like kimchi or sauerkraut, can help your gut stay balanced even through the prescriptions and stress.

Remember to always keep your doctor in the loop anytime you want to make add something into your regimen! Foods and supplements can go a tremendous way to supporting your recovery during and after treatment. I would highly recommend digging into resources, hiring a practitioner that can support you, and finding what works for your life and your budget.

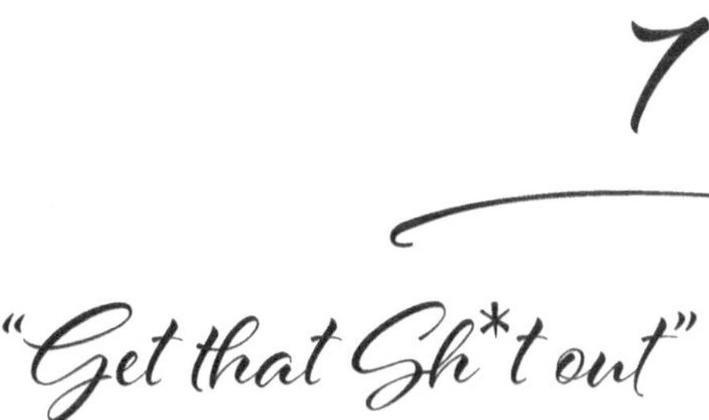

7

"Get that Sh*t out"

Working on gut health day-to-day, I talk about poo all the time with my clients so I think poo puns are punny. Part of my healing journey was dealing with emotional baggage and releasing some things consciously and subconsciously along the way… in a few moments I will talk about emotional constipation, but while we're on the subject, let's discuss physical constipation since it's an important consideration during treatment.

If you are constipated, it can really mess with your whole body. You can reabsorb toxins, experience hormone imbalances, feel pain… it's not fun. You gotta get that sh*t out. Literally! Pooping should be a major priority for you. I've mentioned a few things you may incorporate like probiotics, prunes, and natural laxatives when necessary… but do you know what to look for in *healthy* poop?

Shockingly, many will tell you that if you poop three times a week you aren't constipated. In reality, here is what you want to look for in healthy poo:

- You poo every day a minimum of once. Preferably two or three times.
- You poo within 20-45 minutes of waking up (especially if you

are up and moving within that time).
- Your poo doesn't stink up the whole bathroom.
- You don't see excessive amounts of undigested foods in your poo.
- It's long, not chunky (little balls, chunky poos, or hard and uncomfortable to push is leading to constipation).
- Should be soft but held together.
- It's not a weird color (green, black, yellow etc....) – medium-brown color is normal.
- You don't need coffee to go.

Obviously, some of these things will change during treatment and I wouldn't worry too much as long as you are GOING. But, pull out this list and start monitoring when you are done, because this is important every day!

Emotional constipation

Just like it's important to get literally sh*t out of your body, it's important to deal with the emotional stuff too. To be frank, if you have cancer, you've got to work on your emotional constipation or it will kill you one way or another. Mindset, mentality and emotional health are crucial to our ability to heal and while this is something I'm just now digging into more deeply, I knew enough when getting diagnosed that I needed to address my cancer from a physical, spiritual *and* emotional perspective.

In Chinese medicine they speak of your life force, or chi, as getting "stuck" in different organs and parts of your body. The purpose of acupuncture and herbalism is to stimulate the movement and flow of that chi and to keep things flowing smoothly. Chinese medicine also attributes different emotions with different organs and diseases. For example, if you cannot release grief which is connected to your lungs, you may end up with some sort of disease of the lungs. If you are someone that lives in a lot of fear you may experience problems with your kidneys and so forth.

The Indian Ayurvedic traditions talk about the seven chakras (an area of energy) and this has a lot of correlations with Chinese medicine traditions. Things get stuck. Your chakra is blocked. The energy is not flowing properly in one of them and it affects the whole body, causing disease.

I get it… if you are hearing this for the first time this sounds *totally* cuckoo. I feel you. I was raised in a conservative Christian home where I had to sneak Christian music CDs in the house. (Side note: I recently made a joke with my parents about that. We were sitting at a Celtic Festival listening to some rowdy Celtic music and I said to my Dad, "Hey earlier I told Keegan how I used to have to sneak Christian music into the house. And here we are listing to pagan music and tapping our feet. It must be the devil." My Dad replied, "That never happened," and we both laughed.

We learn, we grow, it's all good. But my point is, if you are coming from a background where energy healing sounds crazy, I understand my friend. But what the heck do you think prayer is? What do you think the laying on of hands is? What do you think the spiritual gift of healing is?

I have experienced enough emotional healing and spiritual events in my life that I am now ON BOARD. My belief is that what the Chinese call chi, the Bible calls the breath of life. When God breathed life into Adam, it was the single differentiating factor that made his body function. We can't see it, we can't feel it, but we know it's there. Why does a heart stop without a major disease in the body? Because the breath of life simply leaves when it's time to go. Why do we have an innate sense of eternity when all we can comprehend is a temporal life and then death? Why does everyone search for purpose if there is none?

Why do we feel that our deepest self is completely distinct from our physical body?

Simply put, it's because we are spiritual beings living in physical clothes. That breath of life is exactly what makes us tick. And because of sin, sadness, trauma, fear, and well... life on earth as human beings... we can shift the energy in our bodies. We can harbor, and stuff things down and refuse to let go of negative experiences and past hurts, and ultimately this can lead to disease...

I think it's a tremendous shame that Christianity has shunned practices like energetic healing and here's why: 20 years ago, yoga was viewed by many as a mystical religious practice. Today, it's widely accepted as something that helps you breathe deeply, and improve your strength, flexibility and mental focus. Anyone with any religion can practice it freely and experience the benefits.

I believe the same to be true for energetic work. Science has flat-out proven that we are made of energy. We are all quite literally vibrating intensely. If you zoom into the microscopic parts of us, we are just a bunch of cells vibrating together in an organized way. Technically, if you moved fast enough, we could walk through each other!

My point is this, energy is real. Energy gets stuck. God created us this way. Of all things, as a Christian, instead of writing it off as voodoo, wouldn't you want other Christians to learn about it and to be the ones offering the healing and the therapies?

If that is too bizarre to think about, just think about this. We have all "vibed" off of someone. We get a sense of that person simply by being near them. While conversation helps to dial it in, it's not really neces-sary. There is an energy that we all emanate and we can transfer and absorb each others energies as well.

Think back to a time when you left a situation where you were talking with someone and you thought to yourself: "Oh my gosh, that was so exhausting. She is so negative and that just took the energy right out of me to even have that conversation". I'm sure you can also think of times when you sat with someone else and left thinking: "That was so refreshing! She just filled me up and I feel so energized just spending time with her."

What radiates from within: sadness, pain, trauma, anger… manifests outwardly to the point where others can sense it. If that's happening person-to-person how much more do you think it's manifesting internally in your own body?

When healing we have to address all the layers of the physical, mental, emotional, spiritual and the energetic fields. I recall when I got sick 25 years ago. I thought the chronic fatigue, fibromyalgia, M.S. and allergies were all physical problems.

I knew there was more healing needed… I kept seeking and worked on my mental game, kept a gratitude journal, spent time in nature and still wasn't were I wanted to be. Then I found biofeedback and energy work and began to put the pieces together.

To heal completely addressing the layers all at once (body, mind , spirit and energy field) by using my Multi- dimensional BRAIN System is faster.

What I figured out is that the brain holds the emotions and memory of sickness and past traumas that contribute to Cancer or illness. These create lesions and take up space in the brain not allowing our soul's truth to shine (why we call it brain-soul). We are a soul with a body, not a body with a soul. The masters in China said we heal in the spaces- (the space in the crevices of the brain, between the heart and lung, between the nerves, between the lymph and the skin, etc.)

All pain is emotional and can be released. Emotions carry a frequency or charge. We have to clear the abuse, memories of the bully in third grade, the abandonment, shame, guilt and grief. When we clear the emotions or past trauma's the person feels lighter and more aligned and they HEAL! COMPLETELY! We are clearing the cellular memory bumps or lesions.

I just love watching people heal, holding space for that journey. I can admit that I would not be doing such deep work with people if I had not had a near death experience myself.

What a gift and teacher our struggles are. Kylene's courage and journey is her gift from God. I know we will observe her power come out more now and this was part of the divine plan for her life.

Healers get to heal themselves and the more powerful the person the bigger the struggle. God Bless!

Louise Swartswalter -creator of the the B.R.A.I.N system

Disease may just be body, mind, spirit and energy out of balance.

Faith

The same is true for our positive thoughts and emotions. When we are brave enough to work through our fears, our angers, our sadness and our traumas, instead of identifying yourself as a victim from those situations, we are able to once and for all release them. This leaves space to experience joy, thankfulness, gratefulness, peace and a newly found freedom.

In the Bible, Jesus says: "Peace I leave with you. My peace I give to you. Not as the world gives, do I give to you. Let not your hearts be troubled, neither let them be afraid." John 14:27

And in John 6:35 he also said: "I am the bread of life, whoever comes to me will never go hungry. And whoever believes in me will never be thirsty."

I feel the need to share these passages with you because without my faith in Jesus Christ as my personal savior, someone who laid down His life for mine and offers me a personal relationship with the creator of the universe, I truly do not know how I would deal with emotionally difficult situations.

Many in the cancer community share that the emotional part is the hardest. The fear during treatment, the fear after treatment that it will come back, and the discouragement and emotional burden of being diagnosed. While of course I experienced many similar emotions, it was my faith that gave me purpose. I knew that God was with me, I knew that people were praying for me to heal, and I knew that whether I liked it or not, God had a plan for this part of my life. I simply needed to be open and willing to receive it.

Faith was the number 1 thing that got me through my treatment. And it's the number 1 thing that keeps me going in life. Sure, emotional resiliency is important, but where does that even come from? My reality cannot be separated from my faith because it is so deeply part of who I am. If this is something you still struggle with: finding purpose, feeling lost, not knowing how your life will look after this, I would encourage you to pick up a Bible and begin reading the book of John. God is here and He loves you. And so do I. There is more to this life than simply being a "good person" and doing your best. You were created, designed lovingly, and given life for a greater purpose.

Transitions

About treatment four, I felt physically that the chemo was done. I didn't really feel like there was much progress being made and I didn't think that I needed the last two treatments. But it was between treatment five and six when I had a major spiritual shift. Let me explain.

Through this entire process, I had been experiencing spiritual downloads: revelations about how I wanted to spend my time when I was cancer-free; how I wanted to host classes in my new home to teach things I love; build stronger relationships with women in my community; and I was trying to be open to whatever lessons God wanted me to learn.

But I tell you what, the biggest lesson happened after chemo session five. I had been acquaintances with a woman for about a year and half, and she was a very negative woman. She thought she was positive, and perhaps in her circle of influence she was in comparison, but no, she was negative. Every time we would get together she would communicate how unhappy she was with every aspect of her life, but she was also afraid to make any dramatic changes. On some level, she was comfortable in her discomfort.

One day, I shared a story with her about how my husband told me to "get over it" once, and how, while that sounds really harsh, it really helped me mentally. I reiterated multiple times during the conversation how I was only saying this in love because I wanted her to be happy. Most of the conversation really surrounded getting her to set boundaries, saying no, and spending some time doing things for herself that made her feel good.

I later found out that I really offended and embarrassed her. Instead of telling me directly, I found this out through a mutual friend. I voluntarily reach out to let her know that if I said anything to hurt or offend her that was not my intention.

Months go by and I posted something on Facebook about personal responsibility and she commented. It wasn't a mean or nasty comment, but I could tell she was still upset with me and hadn't let it go, so I deleted the comment.

Long story short: She saw that I deleted it, reached out to me, and this turned into a day of back and forth messages that culminated in the end of our relationship. I was angry. I was riled up. I was all the feelings.

We had technically both apologized by the end of it but I needed some space from it all. While I still don't feel like I did anything technically wrong, there were some realizations I ultimately needed to come to after some time had passed:

1. Our energy wasn't good together. The separation was a positive thing.
2. It didn't matter whether I was justified or not, whether I intended to hurt her or not, I had. She also had old wounds and traumas and somehow I was triggering them.
3. She was also triggering me and my old traumas too. It would be easy to remain angry and blame her for everything, but taking responsibility means that I don't point all of that out. I just own it and accept my part in her story.

So I thought about that for a few days. It just stayed with me that I needed to reach out one final time for my own emotional healing and resolution, and apologize sincerely for hurting her so that I could close this chapter.

That email went out between chemo session five and six and that is when I spiritually felt like the cancer was gone. I had heard of people experiencing the "knowledge" that their cancer was gone, but I didn't know if I would experience it myself.

I would encourage you to be brave and look internally to discover if there are any past wounds, traumas, relationships or thoughts that need to be freed. When you have cancer you can no longer afford to carry these things with you—they simply become a stressor piled on top of an already full bucket of physical dirt. I do hope that you get to experience this feeling, because it's as if a huge weight is lifted off you in a time when that is a welcome gift.

I don't care if you have been molested, cheated on, divorced, or betrayed. And I can say that with love because I have experienced each of those things in my life. They are not worth holding on to.

Sit with that for just a moment. Those are four of the most horrific things that may happen to you as someone living in the United States. Betrayal. Affairs. Molestation... I repeat: **THOSE EXPERIENCES. ARE. NOT. WORTH. HOLDING. ON. TO.**

They are not worth defining the rest of your life. Your experiences don't define you unless you allow them to. You are a separate person from your experiences, and choosing to define yourself around a moment in time is only hurting you. It doesn't allow you to get revenge. In fact, holding these feelings of anger, resettlement and victimhood hurts no-one other than your own mind, spirit and body.

Every time you rehash a bitter thought, an angry word, or focus on the pain from a previous experience, you pour more salt on the wound and instead of releasing it and allowing it to heal, you let it fester. Festering wounds cause infection. Infection leads to disease, and left unchecked disease leads to death.

Alternatively, if you put honey on the wound by allowing yourself to fully process the grief, the trauma, and the pain and say: "This no longer serves me, I'm willing to forgive. I'm willing to let go. I'm willing to let God help me do this". Then the honey protects the wound from getting infected. It allows the wound to heal. And when the wound heals you develop scar tissue that is stronger than the skin it replaced.

Forgiveness is never about the other person. Often it's hard to forgive because we think it's all about the person who harmed us. Forgiveness is really about you. The person who has been hurt. Forgiveness allows you to release that anger, release that hurt, and it allows YOU to heal. I'm not saying it's easy. In fact, I think forgiveness is one of the most difficult actions you can take.

So here is my challenge to you: Work with your past, hire an energy healer, get acupuncture, pray, read books, do whatever it is that you need to do in your unique story to get that negative sh*t out. And then revel in the freedom that it provides and just wait for the healing to begin.

> "A cheerful heart is good medicine,
> but a crushed spirit dries up the bones."
> Proverbs 17:22

A drop in the bucket

I REALLY LOVE teaching. You know how Enneagram tests are all the rage right now? Well years ago, spiritual gift testing used to periodically go around the churches. I think its super cool and fun anytime you can get an insight into your personality. I mean, it's *way* easier to analyze other people, am I right? But when it comes to yourself—total blindspot.

Patrick and I recently took a free Enneagram, and for all of you who just read that last paragraph and wondered about the results: I'm a 3 and my husband is a 2. I need verbal affirmation and my husband needs a "thank you" here and there after helping the world solve all its problems.

I discovered through the spiritual testing at church that I was a prophet and a teacher. I can see things and explain things and I love to do it. So when I work with my clients, I really enjoy teaching them a little bit about the science behind the process, protocols and why I'm recommending what we do so that they can then internalize it better.

How many times have you been to the doctor or nutritionist, you've been given a pill or a supplement or tea, and you go home and two weeks later you're like: "Wait, why am I taking this? What the heck does this do?" My mission is to empower women to become the facilitators of health in their homes and in order to do that they need to know what's going on. I want them to go from homemakers to healthmakers!

One topic I discuss often with my clients is the "bucket of health". If you've ever read *The 5 Love Languages*, Gary Chapman talks about your love tank and how identifying yours and your spouse's love languages allows you to fill their love tank. We can view health and disease in much the same way.

Our bodies have a tolerance "bucket". And each stressor, whether it be mental, emotional or physical stress, adds up to one drop in the bucket. Your body is designed to self-clean, like a bathtub with an open drain, for example. Stress comes in, your body adjusts, cleans itself out, and empties the bucket. The problem comes in when there are so many stressors that the drain gets clogged. And then the bucket begins to fill up. And eventually, a single drop that seems insignificant and minuscule tips the bucket enough that the drops begin to drain off the side, creating symptoms. The symptoms continue to become more irritating until the bucket tips over and finally you have a dis-ease state in your body.

I think this analogy reminds us that disease does not happen overnight. It takes days, weeks and even years of stressors to accumulate before our bodies can no longer work as efficiently.

This is why taking seemingly small symptoms seriously is important. Things like fatigue, acid reflux, bloating, irregular cycles, PMS, acne... while incredibly common, these are *not* normal and need to be addressed.

When it comes to cancer, often there is a big bucket filled with extra toxic drops. And before I go any further, don't let this section make you feel guilty. There are so many things that come together in order to develop cancer that I don't ever want you thinking: "Oh no, I did this to myself!" No. We do what we can, with the knowledge we have at the time. And much of it is out of our control.

However, once we get into remission, this concept is really important because we want that drain to stay open and that bucket to stay empty! Or as low as possible.

There are many things that fill our bucket including:

- The air we breathe.
- The water we drink.
- The processed foods we eat.
- Body products.
- Medicines.
- Smoking.
- Drinking too much alcohol.
- Poor sleep habits.
- Stressful lifestyle (workaholic, go go go).
- Not enough joy in life (relaxation, laughing, stress relief).
- Not enough movement.
- Too much exercise.
- Home cleaning products.
- Fragrances, wall plug-ins, sprays.

And so much more…

I was joking with someone the other day when they made a comment of "What's killing us?" and I said it's a shorter list to ask, 'What *isn't* killing us?" Funny not funny.

While it's true that we are bombarded with daily stressors in our lives from the food we eat to the water we drink, the homes we live in, the products we choose to use and the air we breathe, the good news is that so much of it is within our control.

Remember, we have pretty big buckets. God designed our body in an amazingly intricate way from our liver to our kidneys to our kick-ass immune systems if we just give it some encouragement. Our body totally knows what to do when it has the right tools and it's really good at it. Our job is to simply be conscientious about the toxic load, so that we can minimize what we have control over and relax about what we don't.

Imagine if over the next year you stopped eating out. You simply gave up soda, processed foods and fast food, and you slowly learned how to cook. Even if it wasn't all organic and perfect, that alone would have an incredibly big impact.

Then let's say you took another step and decided to focus on your skin and body care. You decide to screen everything you're thinking of using or are currently using through the EWG.org website to see what the toxicity rating is and if it's above a level three you ditch it and switch. That too would be a huge step towards maintaining the levels of your bucket.

This sort of transition from toxic to a non-toxic lifestyle is not something that will happen overnight, but any step you take is a good one.

8

You were born for such a time as this

QUEEN ESTHER WAS one of my favorite Bible stories. When I was a kid, we had lots of audio cassette tapes to listen to before we went to bed. I think we had three separate versions of Esther and I probably wore all of them out listening over and over and over again.

Esther was a beautiful Jewish woman, who became the Queen of Persia, and ultimately, through her bravery and faith in God, saved her people from slaughter. When Esther became Queen, she kept her nationality secret at first. Or at least, she didn't blurt out that she was a Jew. When she found out through her cousin Mordecai that her people were in danger, he pleaded for her to go before the King and ask for his mercy. This could mean death for her if she wasn't welcomed into his throne room, but Mordecai replied: "Do not think to yourself that in the King's palace you will escape any more than all the other Jews. For if you keep silent at this time, relief and deliverance will rise for the Jews from another place, but you and your father's house with perish. ***And who knows whether you have not come to the kingdom for such a time as this?***" Esther 4: 13-14

When I was in the throes of research, trying to figure out exactly what treatment I wanted to use and what was available to incorporate into my regimen to keep me strong, a fellow FDN recommended that I reach out to another practitioner.

When I did, she was essentially zero help at all, and after telling me to eat like a rabbit, she said, "You'll be fine! It is really a gift, cancer. You are now really seeing the beauty of this world and small things and people are no longer relevant. It's a teaching moment".

Um. EXCUSE ME?! It's a gift? A teaching moment? RUDE. I immediately unfriended her because I was so frustrated that someone I didn't know very well would have the gall to say something so insensitive.

At the same time, although I felt that her words were unkind, I also knew on some level that they had truth. I knew that this was part of God's plan. I knew that there was a purpose for this. I knew that I would come out the other side learning lessons and having spiritual downloads and major life shifts. But please. Don't tell me just after diagnosis that this is a gift, lady!

So no, I won't tell you that this is a gift, but I will share how intricately purposeful God was in the timing and orchestration of my cancer diagnosis.

I already mentioned that I scrolled back in my phone to discover pictures of the tumor developing at least two years prior to when I saw it. There are stories in the Bible of God taking the "scales" off of people's eyes, or revealing truths at specific times, and I am wholly convinced that this is what He did for me. I didn't *need* to know that I had cancer developing in 2016. In fact, that would have been the absolute wrong time to discover it.

Back in 2016 I was just getting into social media more consistently to develop my online fitness coaching business. This really taught me a lot about social media presence, and how to use it to grow my business. I took that knowledge and used it as I began to shift away from online fitness into wellness, and ultimately into my career as an FDN-P and functional medicine health coach.

Had I not established my social media presence then, I would not have had the support or platform that I did through my treatment.

What really spurred me to become an FDN was a major health crisis in 2015 where I spent two weeks with insomnia, and a non-stop panic attack where I would cry every day, be jumpy and scared at everything. I experienced intrusive thoughts and over all felt legitimately crazy! I didn't know what was happening to me and I went to my doctor twice in that period of time. The second time she wanted to offer me an anti-depressant. I knew I wasn't depressed and I had dipped my toes into the health world just enough to ask her, "Should I get my hormones tested?" "Not if you're still cycling normally, I don't really see any reason to do that" she said. So I left, completely devastated, with no answers, and I remember sitting across from my husband who had taken the day off work, as I held his hand and cried. You see, he had taken several days off work during this time to babysit me and if he couldn't do it, my Mom would come over. I felt like an extreme burden, all the while having no idea why all of a sudden my brain was going crazy and I felt so unlike myself.

It was then that I decided to follow my gut and pursue hormone testing myself. That opened the door for me to begin discovering root causes of dysfunction in my body. I discovered that I had post-menopausal level hormones and was able to get the help I needed to scratch and claw my way out of that scary black hole of fear.

Once stable, I had a voracious appetite to learn more about my body and how I could support it, to keep this from every happening again. I didn't want to just be ok, I wanted to feel great.

This led me to take an online hormone program a year later where I re-tested my hormones and got a lot more information about lifestyle and supplementation. I wanted to know what those ladies knew! One of them was an FDN and I was considering getting some sort of nutrition certification or other health coaching certification to further my education, heal my body, and help other people who needed what I needed.

This ultimately led to me opening my own business, all the while working on my own gut health and hormones. I'm convinced that the two-year period while I was doing all of this work strengthened my body to get through treatment, and potentially even slowed down or stopped the spread of the cancer.

FDN led me to an incredible online community of functional health practitioners organized by J.J. Virgin. This community is where I found my integrative oncologist, my emotional energy coach, and my detox coach. It's also where I developed new friends and received incredible business coaching advice from other like-minded health entrepreneurs. And it's the main impetus behind the writing of this book. I didn't want to be known as "the cancer girl". I didn't want to identify with my disease. I wanted it to be a blip in my life and I didn't really want to talk much about it after that. But someone from this group looked at me and told me I didn't have a choice. This was my platform. And I needed to embrace it.

So you see, God knew that this would happen. He allowed it to happen. But He set me up for success because there was a purpose behind it. I didn't see the tumor until I was healthy enough mentally and physically to survive chemotherapy. I didn't get the diagnosis until I had a community that I was able to reach out to for support and a platform that was available for me to share my journey so that I could encourage others through the process.

I don't know what your purpose will be, or what lessons you will learn. I certainly couldn't have predicted this book on January 8th 2019, when I went into the doctor's office to check on the lump. But I did know as soon as I got the diagnosis that something good would come from it. So I encourage you to hold onto that. Pray, be open, listen to what comes to you through this journey. The purpose is beyond our comprehension. But it is my belief that if you have this diagnosis, then just perhaps, ***you were born for such a time as this.***

9

Spiritual Downloads

I REMEMBER WHEN I started getting into the health world, all the experts and everyone I admired had these amazing morning routines, they would all do deep things like meditate daily, read tons of books and be all Zen.

I admire that, but if you are like me and have a totally ADD brain, meditation is difficult! I mean, there's a big part of me that really wants to have this consistent morning routine that includes devotions, reading, stretching, and walking my dog… And maybe someday I'll get there. But I'm here to encourage you that you do not *have* to meditate or have your life in perfect order to receive spiritual downloads throughout this process.

I would encourage you to pray and pray often. Ask God what it is that He wants you to learn on this journey and ask to be open to the information when it comes. Then just wait. Take walks barefoot and leave your cell phone at home. Take more opportunities to be present and in the moment even when you're alone. Consider meditation, taking time alone, journaling or simply sitting for 5-10 minutes and focusing on deep breathing.

The power of positive thinking

Hope, gratefulness, and positive thinking can become powerful trans-formations all on their own in your life and health. What we think becomes reality. Our thoughts become feelings and feelings become actions and actions manifest outcomes. It's critically important, especially when under the pressure and stress of a cancer diagnosis, to make sure that the majority of our thoughts are positive ones.

If positive thinking is new or difficult for you, then take this opportunity to develop that part of yourself. You won't be perfect. I had my down moments and my crying days too! It may not be an overnight transformation but it's worth the effort.

If you're not used to positive thinking, or find it difficult at this time, it may take some practice but here are some simple strategies to try:

1. Put a rubber band on your wrist. Yes, we're going old school here! If you really need to be snapped out of it (see what I did there...) then take this more dramatic approach: any time you catch yourself thinking, "But what if..." Or, "I can't..." Or anything that you feel is too negative, snap the rubber band. Then immediately rephrase the thought in your mind. For example: "I don't know if I'm strong enough to handle this" turns into "I have survived every challenge so far" or, "Why me?" Turns into, "Why not me? I'm chosen for a purpose".

2. A more gentle and yet still effective process is to begin a gratitude journal. It can be in your phone, on your lap top, or handwritten in a pretty new journal that your purchase for the occasion. You only need to do two things, so it's not too time-consuming. At night before going to bed, write down three things that you are thankful for from that day. When you wake up in the morning, write down three positive things that will happen that day. This is a really effective way to wake up and set your intention for the day by looking for opportunities to be grateful.

3. Surround yourself with positive people. Positive friends, family members, and positive mentors in books etc.…. Surrounding yourself with people that help to encourage you, give you positive sayings, or give you things to look forward to can be tremendously helpful during this process. Conversely, separating yourself from those that drain you mentally and emotionally is just as important. You may have had the capacity to handle it before, but you probably won't now and *you* are your number one priority during this time.

I'm not saying there won't be down days. There certainly are plenty of them throughout this journey. Fear may slip in, fatigue from the treatments, anxiety over the next steps… there's nothing wrong with feeling your emotions, sharing them, and having a good cry. You are not weak for experiencing these things; you're human. But we don't want to wallow in that place. We don't want that to become the new normal.

Looking to the future

You may find yourself asking questions like: "What do I want my life to look like when I'm in remission?" If you haven't already asked that question, I would encourage you to do this. This is where many of my positive thoughts began to focus. I would visualize holding classes in my new home, growing an herb garden (something I've never done), spending time with friends drinking coffee in my new kitchen, and going on a vacation with my husband. Find the thoughts that inspire you and then come back to those regularly during this process.

In fact, take five minutes right now to think about what you want to accomplish when you are cancer-free. Is there anything you can being adding in now? Write down all your dreams and goals that come to mind, no matter how big or small!

____

____

____

____

____

____

____

Netflix

Netflix and chill girl! Yes, Netflix gets its own little headline, that's how much I watched it during treatment. I spent about 48 hours in bed after treatments, excluding some meals and walks outside. So there was a *lot* of watching TV and I want to give you permission that while I'm over here encouraging you to find purpose, and be grateful, it's totally ok to have those days where you completely check out. In fact, you *need* those days. The wonderful thing about TV and movies is that they help you escape from your reality. You can jump into a fairytale world, or a mystery, or a documentary. You can get invested in a 10-season show and I promise you'll have time to finish it all.

Respect your needs during this time, whether it means sleeping, eating, exercising, or just Netflix and chilling. It's OK. Just be aware of your mindset. Are you getting depressed watching too much TV and staying secluded from people? Get on the phone and get together with a friend. But listen to your body and respect what it needs. Sometimes you may be in bed and feel like you have enough energy to go out and do something, and then get up and realize you only felt that good because you were resting.

It's tough to find the balance between pushing yourself to stay engaged and listening to what you need without becoming a couch potato. The balance is different for everyone so just be kind with yourself.

Movement

One of the best things you can do for your mindset and body is to get outside and take walks. Thankfully, I was able to do this every day throughout treatment, although the duration and number of walks would vary depending on how I felt. I always made an effort to get outside a few times each day. Getting sun exposure on our skin and in our eyes not only improves your mood, but it helps with your circadian rhythm, immune system and so much more. This is not something to skimp on during treatment if at all possible. Many spiritual downloads may come during this time. I know many of my best ideas spark when I'm out walking the dog, praying, absorbing the sun and appreciating the outdoors!

While you need to be careful with sun exposure because of the chemotherapy, everyone is different. I just got really tan and had blotchy, uneven skin tone from the sun exposure, but some people may get a rash reaction due to the medication. Be careful, especially for the first 72 hours after treatments, and use an umbrella or cover up if that's a concern but don't stop going outside!!

Sunscreen: I do not advise wearing sunscreen since you will not get the benefits from the sun if you do. I always recommend getting as much sun naturally as you can before your body tells you it's time to be done. Then it's time to cover up, get inside, and protect your skin.

Many sunscreens contain chemicals that soak through your skin and into your bloodstream. If we are concerned about the effect these sunscreens are having on the coral reefs, how much more should we be concerned about what they are doing to our cancer fatigued bodies!

For more information on the benefits of sun absorption see: Wise Traditions podcast #183 - Is sunscreen okay to use? Also see the book: *Embrace the Sun* by Marc Sorenson

For chemical free sunscreen that is so clean you could eat it see: www.3rdrockessentials.com and use code TINYFITDIVA for a discount!

You can take the idea of getting outside a step further by finding a place that you can walk barefoot on the ground. No, not on concrete or asphalt, but actually on the ground in grass or dirt. This is called "grounding" and it helps you to reconnect with the earth's natural magnetic frequencies and energies. If you can't do this, simply getting to a place where you can be more surrounded by nature is also helpful and can be very relaxing emotionally.

About halfway through treatment I was able to begin Pilates classes. I used to lift weights, and I started again once treatment was over, but I knew that that is a stressor on the body and wanted to be conscientious about the amount of stressors I was exposed to during treatment. Not to mention I was tired and immune-compromised. Each individual will respond differently. Some are able to work-out through treatment, some can only walk, and some can do yoga or Pilates. There are so many variables based on your fitness capacity prior to treatment, and your reaction to the treatment. Don't beat yourself up if you aren't able to do the same things you are used to.

It was hard for me to see my body change and not be able to do all the things I really enjoyed regularly. But getting back into a work-out setting, even though it was much more gentle, helped boost my mood tremendously and made me feel like I was getting back to my regular life.

Find what works for you and what feels good, and then be careful not to push yourself too hard! Once treatment is over, you can build yourself right back up!

Exercise is safe and effective both during and after most types of cancer treatment, and should therefore be included as an integral part of an individual's cancer care plan. More than two decades of research support a link between a physically active lifestyle and positive physiological and psychological changes in cancer survivors. These include improvements in $VO_{2\,max}$, which in turn improve heart and lung function and promote a healthy blood pressure, blood volume, and gas exchange. In addition, improvements in quality of life, muscular strength and endurance, fatigue reduction, anxiety, depression, body image, immune function and emotional well-being have been reported. The type and degree of the physiological responses is dependent on the type and dose of exercise.

Physical Activity Guidelines

There are a number of recommendations for physical activity, based largely on observational epidemiologic research linking exercise and cancer risk. The most current recommendations for prevention and survival come from the World Cancer Research Fund, American Institute for Cancer Research, American Cancer Society, and American College of Sports Medicine. More research has been provided discussing benefits of exercise with a risk reduction in cancer diagnosis. Little research, however, has been done on the benefits of exercise with cancer survivorship, so current recommendations reflect prevention guidelines with some treatment- and disease-specific modifications. Both guidelines include moderate physical activity (such as a brisk walk) for at least 30 minutes every day, as well as strength training and stretching of major muscle groups a minimum of 2 days each week.

Ideally, for an individual undergoing cancer treatment, the prescription will include a whole-body workout that targets all the major muscle groups. The overall goal of the exercise program should be to minimize the general de-conditioning that often results from cancer treatment so that the cancer treatments are better tolerated. In general, the exercise prescription should include a slow progression and demonstrate adaptability to changes in the patient's health status, which frequently change from day-to-day during treatment.

Each exercise training session should consist of the following components:

- **Warm up:** Each session should begin with a 5- to 10-minute warm-up that stimulates blood flow to the working muscles. Warm-up activities may include walking or jogging to increase the body temperature and other physiologic responses, as well as decrease the chance of injury. Warm-up activities are also important to help ensure that the muscles and cardiovascular system are prepared for the activities to come in the training session.

- **Aerobic Component:** During the aerobic component of exercise, it is important to frequently monitor blood pressure and heart rate. If the patient is on a medication that effects heart rate, the Borg Scale of Exertion may be used to monitor intensity. Based on this scale, a light-to-moderate intensity (RPE of 11 to 14) should be encouraged. If dizziness, nausea, or chest pain occurs, all exercise should be stopped. Frequent short breaks are sometimes encouraged to accommodate therapy-related fatigue.

- **Resistance Training:** The type of resistance exercise performed will depend on the patient's range of motion, tissue removal, and wound healing. ACSM recommends at least 48 hours of rest between each resistance training session. Therefore, it may be advisable to plan a whole-body approach to resistance training, where all major muscle groups are targeted in one day. If the patient is unwilling or unable to participate in traditional modes of strength training, Yoga or Pilates may serve as an alternative form of strength exercise.

-Karen Wonders, Ph.D., FACSM, Executive Director of Maple Tree Cancer Alliance

10
____

Clean up your environment

MY MOM IS a babe. A total hottie. In the 70s when she met my Dad she was the gorgeous girl wearing wide leg pants, shoulder-length straight hair parted down the middle, and she was so naturally beautiful that she never had to wear a stitch of makeup. My Dad was a national athlete in gymnastics and all the girls wanted to date him, but my Mom caught his eye as the prettiest incoming freshman in the year book. True story.

I love that my Mom never got into makeup for so many reasons. One, she wasn't focused on vanity but frankly, she never had to be. As I have grown up and come to realize however, another reason I'm so glad she never got into makeup is because of all the heavy metals and chemical exposures typical cosmetics can provide.

What we put on our skin gets absorbed into the bloodstream in less than 30 seconds. We now know that toxic load is a major contributing factor to cancer, and that environmental chemicals, heavy metals and other products are becoming more linked to the development of cancer cells and immune system suppression.

A wide variety of metals and other contaminants like lead, mercury, and aluminum are often in makeups you may wear daily including lipstick and eyeliners. Contaminants are not listed directly on the label so it's important to be aware and look for cosmetic companies that do rigorous testing and are committed to creating safe products. Learn more at www.safecosmetics.org

You may have been hearing a lot about glyphosate, the pesticide used in weed killers and how exposure is being linked (through several legal cases) to cancer development.

"Well, I don't work on a farm, I'm not bathing in the stuff," you think. But glyphosate is the largest pesticide used in the world according to EWG.org, and while you may think you're making healthy choices by feeding yourself or your children oats or cereals in the morning, both of those are soaked in glyphosate. In fact, as recent as June 2019, EWG shared an article stating: "Two rounds of laboratory tests commissioned by EWG found glyphosate in nearly every sample of oat-based cereal and other breakfast products at levels higher than what EWG scientists consider protective for children's health..."

This can and should be shocking. Not only are there scientific studies proving that this disrupts your microbiome (a problem in and of itself) but now we have evidence that the amount we are exposed to in one serving of "healthy" breakfast cereals is unsafe. And let's be honest, who measures a serving of cereal? You get exposed at breakfast, and then have a sandwich at lunch with whole-wheat toast, and then maybe you do some gardening a bit later in the day and spray some weed killer on those pesky dandelions and BOOM. You are exposed to a great deal more than your body can handle.

Regardless of where you are on your journey before, during or after a cancer diagnosis, detoxifying your life and environment should be of the utmost priority. Now, I am not an expert on this subject so I will simply share some of the basic information I have and then point you in the direction of other resources that continue to guide you on this journey.

And I'll be honest, it is a journey. I'm still learning and making changes one by one in my own life and I've been doing this for years! No one is going to read this book, wake up the next morning, sell their home and move to the woods. While that would be amazing, it's simply not practical for most of us. So, while you are beginning to learn and make healthy swaps in your home and life environment, don't forget the importance of nutrition to support your body by providing you the nutrients needed to boost your immune system, and assisting in toxin clean up and liver support.

So what exposes us to environmental toxins?

Pesticides

Enough already said! See above!

Utilize EWG.org as a resource and look at their articles on glyphosate exposure. Switch from processed cereals to homemade breakfast and look for organic lawn care options.

Heavy metals

These include lead, mercury, aluminum, zinc, chromium and iron.

Most common exposures:

- lipstick
- water
- anti-perspirant
- cookware
- some dinnerware
- cigarette smoke
- metal fillings that include mercury. These give off gasses in

your mouth and with your gums right there it can go straight into your blood stream and your brain. This does not just happen when you get the fillings put in. It has been shown that even the scraping of a filling with a metal dental tool during a cleaning can cause the filling to off-gas.

Most dentists will tell you that they can remove mercury fillings, but only some (biological/holistic dentists) will do it safely. This requires a process where you are breathing clean air so that you don't get exposed to more mercury as it's being removed, and a physical block (a dental dam) to keep you from ingesting it. The dentist may also use binders which help mop up heavy metals. These are substances like activated charcoal, pectasol C, and bentonite clay. You can look for a dentist that is SMART certified and have a discussion with them prior to the treatment to make sure you are comfortable with their safety procedures and them as a provider.

Take an assessment of what on this list may be your most common exposure, and evaluate where you might like to begin researching swaps.

Deodorant and Antiperspirants

Let me tell you a traumatic story about my childhood. Around puberty, I started sweating. Not like a normal, hey I just ran around the block and I'm misting sweat, but a full-throttle armpit shower all day, every day. I was so embarrassed. I would wear sweaters over my T-shirts and I'd put feminine pads under my armpits stuck to my shirt, whatever it took to hide the fact that there were massive pit puddles *every single day*. Now, I have no idea how long this went on because in kid-world time slows down and everything takes forever. It seemed like years.

One day, my Mom was heading to the doctor and I said "Hey can you ask about this" and she came home with a prescription deodorant that stopped the sweat flow immediately.

I was like, "THAT'S ALL I NEEDED TO DO?! I'm a normal child again." Now looking back I'm thinking, "What the heck was going on in my body that I was sweating that much?", and, "Oh man, what toxins were clogging my pores so badly that I didn't sweat at ALL?!"

I probably used that deodorant for a few years before experimenting with just switching to over-the-counter antiperspirant. But I was so nervous I always looked for the *real* antiperspirant, the high percentage. But do you know what the active ingredient for antiperspirant is? Aluminum. Yup, get your daily dose of heavy metal right there in your armpit where your lymph nodes are waiting to mop it right up.

What really alarmed me and made me look into switching was when I discovered that aluminum was associated with Alzheimer's disease. I was like no thank you, I'm done, I'm out, I'll find another way. It took me a long time to switch to a "clean" aluminum-free deodorant but once I did I've never looked back!

One thing I tell my clients is that everyone is biologically and chemically different. A brand that works well for me, may not work the same for you. That's why I'm providing a list of several below to get you started!

www.primalpitpaste.com

www.primallypure.com

www.nativecos.com

Be aware that aluminum is not the only thing lurking in deodorants, so find a conscientious brand and read labels. Remember, just like your food, you want your deodorant to be made from real ingredients too!

Cosmetics and skincare

It took me *forever* to fully commit to safer skincare and makeup. Not because I didn't care, but because I really wanted to find something that actually worked and performed on the same level as all the conventional brands, without being filled with heavy metals, chemicals, and hormone disruptors.

You'll want to look for brands that commit to eliminating certain ingredients like phthalates, formaldehyde, sulfates and triclosan.

Raise your hand if you have ever tried Mary Kay's eye makeup remover? Totally. It's amazing. I was sure I would never ever switch because it was legit the best. Then I found Beautycounter and made the switch. By the way, their eye-makeup remover wipes score a 1 on the EWG rating–that's the best!

Eventually I found three brands that I love for skincare and I mix and match them depending on what I want:

BeautyCounter: www.beautycounter.com/kyleneterhune

Yep, I use them *so* much I signed up as an advocate! I got hooked on their daily shampoo and conditioner. Seriously, that's all I would commit to at first. Eventually I tried their skincare and now I love and use so many products, including a lotion, eye-makeup remover, skincare and makeup daily!

Crunchi: www.crunchi.com/stephaniellacuna

This is an amazing brand and my girlfriend just happens to sell it so if you choose to try them out please support her! I absolutely *love* their foundation. It smells like vanilla!

Jane Iredale www.janiredale.com

Yet another more conscious brand. I love their full-coverage liquid foundation and often mix it with others for the perfect color or blend.

the *never* list™

WHEN FORMULATING OUR PRODUCTS, WE PROHIBIT THE USE OF OVER 1,500 HARMFUL OR QUESTIONABLE INGREDIENTS.

Benzalkonium chloride · BHA and BHT · Coal tar · Ethylenediaminetetraacetic acid (EDTA) · Ethanolamines (MEA/DEA/TEA) · Formaldehyde · Hydroquinone · Methylisothiazolinone and methylchloroisothiazolinone · Oxybenzone · Parabens (methyl-, isobutyl-, propyl- and others) · Phthalates · Polyethylene glycol (PEG compounds) · Retinyl palmitate and Retinol (Vitamin A) · Sodium lauryl sulfate and Sodium laureth sulfate (SLS and SLES) · Synthetic flavor or fragrance · Toluene · Triclosan and Triclocarban

Beautycounter's never list

And that's just a tiny portion! Beautycounter actually refuses to use over 1500 questionable ingredients. They are constantly utilizing the latest research, and sometimes even commission their own studies when they can't get enough information on an ingredient.

In addition, they created their own definition of the word "safe" since they advertise their products as safer skincare. I love their definition because they clarify that natural products aren't always safe, and synthetic isn't always dangerous. They commit to rigorous testing, the latest research, and as part of the environmental working groups partnership, they also fall under the European Union's standards of cosmetics.

This is just one of many companies following the consumer demand for safer, cleaner skin care and makeup products. Do your research, try a few products out, and find what works best for you!

As much as I love Beautycounter, no brand does everything perfectly and each brand has their strengths and weakness so as you can see I sometimes mix and match brands based on what I need. You can too!

Junk food

I was trying to decide how to title this one because even "health" foods can be a concern like oats, whole wheat, cereal, snack bars etc. Junk food, fake food, processed food, however you'd like to look at it, these all expose us to pesticides, chemicals, food dyes, synthetic ingredients, and sugars that impact our detoxification ability, metabolism, cravings, weight, brain, and immune system.

Begin making the switch to homemade meals with a focus on produce daily. The more organic you can manage the better and I would argue it's not that expensive.

I had this conversation with my husband recently and I said, "You know, if we stopped buying the paleo junk food and just focused on the organic produce our grocery bill would go down".

Every diet has its own version of junk food!! No matter how healthy it is. Of course, that's not to say that you can't treat yourself with a fair trade dark chocolate bar, or some dairy-free ice cream, or whatever it is for you. But the pre-made organic, gluten-free snack foods... that's where the cost of your grocery bill goes up! If the majority of your cart is filled with organic produce and the rest is some high quality meat, beans, etc... You may notice that your grocery bill remains stable or actually drops.

If you find that it increases and makes your grocery budget uncomfortable, you may look into some options like Costco, organic frozen veggies or imperfect organic produce shipped to your door like Misfits Market and Imperfect Produce brands. This provides several options for getting organic produce in bulk or at a discounted rate.

Another consideration is the EWG's annual list, the "Dirty Dozen and the Clean Fifteen". This will help you prioritize which produce to spend the extra money on for organic in order to avoid the heavy pesticide exposure.

As of 2019, the <u>EWG.org</u> Dirty Dozen and Clean 15 list is:

Dirty dozen 2019:	***Clean 15 2019:***
Strawberries	Avocados
Spinach	Sweet Corn
Kale	Pineapple
Nectarines	Sweet Peas (frozen)
Apples	Onions
Grapes	Papaya
Peaches	Eggplant
Cherries	Asparagus
Pears	Kiwi
Tomatoes	Cabbage
Celery	Cauliflower
Potatoes	Cantaloupe
	Broccoli
	Mushrooms
	Honeydew Melon

This list changes each year so be sure to get an updated list!

Don't have the time, or energy, to cook? Try a meal delivery service like MetabolicMeals.com or Freshly.com—you can read all the ingredients for each meal before buying and you can choose how many meals you'd like to order per week.

My suggestion is to do your best, and just commit to continue learning along the way. Don't forget the resources chapter where you can find amazing bloggers, books, and companies to support this new healthy you!

Sugar

Yes, I just talked about food, but sugar deserves its own paragraph because there is some debate on the role that sugar plays in the development of cancer.

In 1931, Dr. Warburg discovered that cancerous tumors prefer sugar as fuel. This is argued in the conventional oncology world today, even while the primary method of diagnosing active tumors is by placing radioactive sugar into the patient and then taking a picture through the PET scan. The whole concept of a PET scan is that the tumor, or active cancer cells, soak up the sugar making it light up on the scan. When a PET comes back clear, it's because the cancer cells are dead or inactive and no longer soak up the sugar injected into the patient.

Whether you come to agree that sugar is fuel for cancer cells or not, at a minimum we know that sugar is inflammatory, causes weight gain, is used excessively in the average American diet, and has a negative impact on blood sugar stability.

I recommend avoiding processed sugar which is stripped of all nutrition and start choosing less processed and more nutrient-dense alternatives like pure maple syrup, raw honey, and dates. If you are looking for a specific recipe to make that would follow these guidelines, simply Google whatever you are looking for with the word "paleo" in front of it and someone somewhere will have come up with a recipe for you!

Try this amazing chickpea brownie recipe!

Ingredients

1 (15 oz) can of chickpeas/garbanzo beans, drained and rinsed
1/4 cup of grass-fed butter (or extra virgin coconut oil)
2 large eggs
1/2 cup of maple syrup
1/3 cup of unsweetened cocoa powder
1/2 tsp baking powder
1 pinch sea salt
1/4 cup of Enjoy Life mini chocolate chips

Directions

- Preheat oven to 350 degrees.
- Line a 9×9 inch baking pan with parchment paper and set aside.
- Place the chickpeas, butter, eggs, maple syrup, vanilla, cocoa powder, baking powder and salt in a food processor. Cover, and blend until smooth.
- Add the chocolate chips and mix by hand until combined.
- Spread the batter evenly into the prepared pan.
- Bake for 25-28 minutes or until a toothpick inserted into the center of brownies comes out clean.
- Cut into squares and leave to cool. Use powdered sugar to decorate with fun patterns for any occasion.

NOTE

These brownies crumble easily so they do better if you let them cool and place them in the refrigerator for a while. It makes them more fudgy and easier to handle! My family *loves* this recipe!

Mold and impure air

The air inside of our homes is often way more contaminated that the air outside. One of the main contaminants that can cause major toxic load is mold exposure. If you live in an older home, have experienced leaks, see bubbles in the drywall, or smell something musty, you may want to get a qualified remediation specialist to check it out.

This is something we often think isn't a problem unless we can *see* it. We think if we don't see green or black mold growing on the wall or tiles it must not be there. But often it can be lurking on the beams of the home, in the ceiling, or behind walls causing all sorts of chronic inflammation in your body.

This is something that my family is currently digging into more; the other thing to think about with mold and toxins is old carpet that has been the place of several animal accidents. My son has been getting sick for the past few years as soon as he gets back to school. He catches strep or some virus going around and then gets so sick he once missed the first few weeks one semester.

Obviously this is a problem, and we have tried everything. We have taken him to the ER, we have run my gut labs on him (which brought up a lot of issues we were able to address), we have occasionally tried antibiotics only to find that they typically make him feel worse in the long run, and we have tried probiotic therapy, supplements, and of course we eat really healthy foods.

So we simply could not understand why his immune system is so weak and suppressed that he cannot seem to recover from normal childhood exposure to illness. Just this year we began to turn our thoughts to mold.

A few years ago, our clothes washer leaked so badly that there were chunks of the drywall falling off the ceiling below. We don't have much carpet in our home but we do have some in the bedrooms and our lovely sweet dog has used Keegan's room as a toilet many times.

When Patrick and I began discussing this, I decided to experiment with Keegan as if we knew it was mold toxicity. One night I gave Keegan a binder (a supplement that assists in binding toxins and flushing them out of your system) and then had him sleep downstairs on the couch away from his bedroom. He woke up feeling good so I think we are on to something!

There is a lot to consider with mold toxicity including who you have come to check it out.

You want to find a company that'll not expose you to more mold during the process and who will test and remediate safely. This in itself is a whole separate book (one that I'm sure has been written by a qualified building biologist).

I would recommend checking out my friend, who was also exposed to mold and did all the research too. She has compiled a list of resources at www.zestyginger.com/moldy

Regardless of mold exposure, it's wise to invest in a quality air purifier. We personally like and use www.airoasis.com. For our new home we purchased the version that connects directly to the HVAC systems purifying the air as it circulates. Cool huh! If you don't want to start there, or if you live in an apartment, you can always get a smaller unit or a room to room unit. Their Air Angel is nice because it works for a bedroom, is small enough to travel and take to hotel rooms, and even has a charger switch that allows you to use it in a car!

You may think you don't need to worry about your car, but I just drove a rental car that had some major air freshener sprayed in it or put in one of the vents right before I started driving it and it was a problem!

You may notice through this process that you become more chemically sensitive. Remember that toxic load we spoke about earlier? That bucket that needs to be drained? Chemotherapy is filling up that bucket and things like chemical sensitivities are reactions that you may begin to experience as a result. This doesn't mean there is anything wrong with you, and it may even go away eventually. But things like a VogMask or an air purifier can go a long way if you find out that this is something that applies to you. A Vogmask is a mask that helps filter air particles, odors, and contaminants. It uses a carbon filter, and an exhalation valve to make using it as effective and comfortable as possible. This is the brand I use and I pull it out whenever I travel to wear on the plane.

Impure water

I grew up thinking you were a snob if you didn't drink tap water. But now I think, if you want to live a healthy life you need to avoid it like the plague! Tap water can be a source of chlorine, synthetic fluoride (the form that is added to the water, not the naturally occurring mineral), parasites like giardia, and trace molecules of leftover prescriptions and pharmaceuticals. NO thank you!

To find out more about your local tap water go to this website: www. ewg.org/tapwater

Even "purified" water often... isn't. For example, I believed that my refrigerator filter was ok for years until I realized that at minimum it wasn't filtering the fluoride out of my water.

For more information on water purification and the problem with fluoride see: www.hiddencauseofacne.com

Many filters like Pur or Brita, simply don't filter some of the major contaminants and while they are a step above tap water, they are still many steps below the kind of water that is most beneficial for our bodies.

If possible, spring water is the best. Naturally purified through our earth's filtration system and mineralized with spring rocks, this water brings the most natural form of purified water to your body.

But living in today's world, it's tough to find a spring, capture your own water, and maintain this homestead habit... what you can do is install a reverse osmosis system that includes a remineralizer. Reverse osmosis purifies the water so much that it even strips it of the beneficial minerals. We don't want that, so you do want the remineralized step! I personally use this brand: Ispring reverse osmosis with remineralization (see resource notes in the back).

Don't want to install a whole unit? You can try an on-counter water filtration system like Berkey or Aqua Tru.

Home building products

You may find, as I did, that you seem to be more chemically sensitive after treatment than you were before. This may simply be that your body now has the freedom to mount an immune system reaction to invaders and is going to more loudly express itself, or it may be something that calms down as you begin to detoxify from treatments.

Regardless, home building products off-gas chemicals that you may want to be aware of, especially if, like us, you are building a new home or moving.

Some top offenders are non-hardwood cabinets, carpet, paint, and vinyl flooring.

We recently made the decision to avoid vinyl planks in our basement and go with polished concrete and hardwood. We were pleasantly surprised to find out that this actually saved us money instead of being more expensive.

Knowing is half the battle because then you can take steps to control what's within your power to control. A great resource would be a website like www.greenbuildingsupply.com.

Overuse of antibiotics and NSAIDS

You might be surprised to see antibiotics under environmental toxins, but I wanted to throw this in here simply because a disruption in your gut microbiome can have dramatic impact on your immune system and your body's ability to defend itself against inflammation or foreign invaders.

Within the first year or so of marriage, I experienced three UTI's (urinary tract infections) all of which I took antibiotics for. Looking back, I think this was part of the stress cascade that eventually tipped over my health bucket!

We all know that antibiotics don't discriminate. While they can be lifesaving and crucial under the right circumstances, they kill the good *and* bad bacteria and are often used too frequently. We need those good bacteria to keep our immune system, energy, brain, hormones and digestion functioning well!

Many, if not most, of my clients who come to me with chronic gut complaints have previously been exposed to many rounds of harsh antibiotics in addition to a few stressful life situations, creating the perfect environment for chronic inflammation and symptom expression.

This is certainly not something you can change in your medical history, but it is something you can be aware of in your decisions moving forward.

Home cleaning products

We all want our laundry whiter than white, our countertops sparkling, our toilets cleaned and our floors shined... but at what cost? The most popular brands of cleaning products are ones that include chemicals that are poisonous if ingested. But for some reason we don't think twice about wearing them and breathing them in every day!

Even the American Lung Association admits that many cleaning supplies can cause reactions of irritation or even serious health problems including cancer.

There are a few companies out there committed to helping your home shine without the chemicals. Here are a few:

Norwex: www.courtneyhemperly.norwex.biz

Their microfiber cloths are UHMAAAAAYZING. The silver threads woven throughout make them antibacterial and there are some pretty fascinating YouTube videos demonstrating how well they mop up raw meat germs.

My green fills: www.mygreenfills.com

For all your laundry needs! I really love this brand and just recently began to use it. The ingredients list is very short, and very clean. If you choose the scented version, it's all essential oils. If you need a hypoallergenic version they provide a non-scented option as well!

Fragrances

One final environmental toxin I wanted to mention is fragrances, which includes air fresheners, wall plugs-ins, scented candles and also perfume. These all contain synthetic compounds, chemicals, and hormone disruptors. Like I mentioned under home building products, you may find that you are more sensitive and experience headaches or inflammation simply from smelling fake smells.

But don't fret, if you are a candle lover, here are some safer alternatives:

- Meyers Clean Day Candles
- Beeswax candles
- Terralite candles

Make the switch by throwing away toxic products like Febreeze, lotions and other products made with fake, or strong, scents and switch to natural products scented with oils or extracts.

Perfume is another consideration and I hate to be "that person", but even if it doesn't bother you it probably bothers me (the people around you breathing it). Whether or not you notice a headache coming on from wearing it, most perfumes are made from synthetic chemicals and fake fragrances and it's wise to switch to more natural options like essential oil blends, or nothing at all!

Keep in mind, this list isn't here to scare you or overwhelm you! There's almost no way unless you are a multi-billionaire that you can construct a life *completely* void of toxins. But being aware is the number one step! From there, you can commit to continually learning and making changes one at a time with the things you are able to control. This will help you to support your body's ability to detoxify naturally, and regularly empty the toxicity bucket.

11

Additional Considerations

I AM THE *worst* packer. I've improved a lot over the past few years since my travel has also increased, but this is how it goes:

"What if I forget something? OK, how many days will I be there? What activities are we doing? What's the weather like? What shoes will go with this outfit? Should I bring my workout clothes? Will I need a sweater?" Ohhhh the pain. The agony. The indecision I have!

And then there are all the pertinent details like contact lenses, solution, and of course, the contacts case which I have definitely forgotten before. Don't worry—while it's not the *best* solution, you can use hotel glasses and submerge your contacts overnight. HA! At least I make it work.

This chapter is like packing for me. There is *so much* to cover when you're discussing cancer, and I just don't want to miss any of it! This is not a scientific book, and I'm not a doctor, but as someone who has personally experienced this terrible disease and also happen to know all of these different lifestyle tools we can utilize, I feel obligated (and honored) to share them with you! At a minimum I can touch on the big picture and guide you to the experts.

I didn't really feel like EMF exposure, Epstein-Barr virus, or budget considerations really fit anywhere else in the book, so I'm packing them in this chapter in a nice little carry on. So buckle up! We have three more things to consider.

EMF

Stop it. Stop it right now. I see you rolling your eyes. You have either heard of EMF exposure and think it's a bunch of hooey, or this is totally new to you and you are like, what the heck is EMF?

I get it, I was totally the same way. Even when you know about it, it's difficult to accept. EMF stands for Electric and Magnetic Fields. This is a form of invisible energy (or radiation) that we are exposed to daily. Why do we care? Because not only has our exposure increased (like glyphosate) but it has also changed in the type of exposure and health dangers associated with it.

Your main exposures are your lap top, cell phone, WI-FI and TV, but you also get different exposures from cell towers, smart meters, baby monitors, Bluetooth and more.

Dr. Mercola, creator of the largest health website in the world, claims that EMFs are the cigarettes of the 21st century. While many health organizations claim that EMFs do not have any known negative effects, many individuals can identify sensitivities to it and find relief when exposure is limited.

One of my favorite food bloggers, Elana Amsterdam, has celiac disease and Multiple Sclerosis. She lives a healthy lifestyle, and uses food as part of that, thus creating the blog www.elanspantry.com and sharing delicious, healthy recipes. A few years ago, when she remodeled her home, using as many green options as she could, she was unaware of EMFs and so everything they did was wireless.

Within two years, she was in the hospital with an MS flare up with symptoms worse than they had been in the past. Ultimately, she discovered building biology and EMF information and removed all the wireless technology from her home and has noticed tremendous benefits.

You can read her story here: elanaspantry.com/green-house-almost-killed

She also has more articles on her website about EMF and how to begin protecting yourself.

Some really simple steps that you can take to limit your exposure today are:

- Shutting the WI-FI off in your home at night.
- Stop wearing a Fitbit or tracker that is constantly emitting WI-FI or Bluetooth.
- Don't hold your phone up to your ear when making calls; use earbuds or put it on speaker.
- When carrying your phone around or when listening to podcasts, put it in airplane mode.
- Keep your phone out of your bedroom, or put it on airplane mode if you have to.
- Find EMF blocking stickers to put on your lap top, phones, and TVs to limit exposure when in use.

There has been no definitive connection between cancer and EMF exposure, but I would throw this in to the toxic bucket. When those with autoimmune disease react to something, they act as a canary in the coal mine for the rest of us. Just because we may not react the same way, doesn't mean the exposure is a healthy thing. I don't know about you, but the diagnosis and treatment of cancer raised my personal dedication to discovering potential toxic exposure and doing my best to eliminate it!

You can find more EMF resources in the back of this book.

p.s. If you have trouble sleeping, I would seriously look into your EMF exposure. What tech do you have in your bedroom at night?

Epstein-Barr Virus (EBV)

Research research research. When I was diagnosed, I was reading ALL. THE.THINGS. Trying to discover what treatment was best, what diet should I follow? What the heck contributed to this disease?

It wasn't long before Epstein-Barr Virus showed up as a known connection to the development of Hodgkin's. Luckily, I had already met the leading expert in this virus, Kasia Kines, so I knew where to go for answers. EBV is a herpes virus that is more commonly known as the cause of mononucleosis (mono). Most of the time this virus is acute (short term) and once the body has dealt with it, it's not a problem. But for some, EBV becomes a chronic problem reactivated with specific triggers.

Kasia immediately recommended that I get tested to see if I was someone that had chronic EBV. Check out Kasia's website www.ebvhelp. com for resources on exactly what markers you need to see on your lab, and how to read them. If you can get your doctor to test, they will often leave one or two critical markers out which can then just be interpreted as "yes, you have, at some point in your life, had this virus" instead of being able to identify if it's currently active.

I was able to get the labs done and ironically enough, discovered that when I tested I was in the middle of a reactivation. Since this was in the first quarter of 2019 while I was still going through diagnosis, staging and research, it made sense. EBV is primarily triggered by stress.

An estimated 15% of global cancer burden can be linked to oncogenic tumor viruses like Epstein-Bar Virus (EBV). EBV is one of the viruses that is suspected to be involved in early stages of tumorigenesis of Hodgkin's and non-Hodgkin's Lymphoma.

Medical literature is very clear that EBV is oncogenic (causing tumor development). This can happen when EBV-infected B cells continue cloning, acquire oncogenic mutations and become neoplastic.

Epstein-Barr Virus (EBV) can also lead to cancer via citrullination of proteins. It is the only virus that causes citrullination. Citrullination is the conversion of one amino acid arginine in a protein into another amino acid citrulline. While citrullination seems to be a physiologically important process, it has been associated with a number of autoimmune disorders and even cancer.

Other than Hodgkin's lymphoma, other types of cancer that are either caused of associated with EBV are: Burkitt's Lymphoma, Pediatric non-Hodgkin's Lymphoma, Cutaneous Lymphoma, Nasopharyngeal Carcinoma, Post-Transplant Lymphoproliferative Disorder, Gastric Lymphoepithelial Carcinoma, B cell, NK/T Cell Tumors or Lymphoma, Angioimmunoblastic T cell Lymphoma, Leiomyosarcoma, Papillary Thyroid Carcinoma, and Malignant Lymphoma of the Thyroid.

In addition, up to 18% of all stomach cancer has been linked to EBV. More studies now also show a link between colorectal and even breast cancer and EBV.

Needless to say, this aggressive and smart virus needs much more attention than we give it.

Dr. Kasia Kines
Doctor of Clinical Nutrition
Author of Amazon best-seller The Epstein-Barr Virus Solution.

This can include mental stress, physical stress and emotional stress. Foods can also trigger it, as well as exposure to mold and other stressors. These same things can negatively impact your hormones as well and stress and suppress the immune system. Stress + suppressed immune system + EBV and you have disease risk. EBV is connected to the development of Hodgkin's in 40 per cent of cases so it's nothing to be ignored.

While I may never know exactly what caused my the development of cancer in my body, you could write a list of potential factors that *I know* I have been exposed to in my personal history:

- Nuclear radiation (lived by a nuclear power plant for 18 years - google Miamisburg Mound Laboratories Leak)
- Frequent antibiotic use
- Birth control medication
- Terrible diet in my late teens and early 20s
- Low sex hormones
- High stress
- EBV
- Aluminum
- EMFs
- Fragrances

I must be very careful in my words here because I do NOT EVER mean to implicate that cancer is your fault. EVER. Some people get it and some people don't. In the same way that two people with the same diet and lifestyle can live very different lives, one becoming sick and another in perfect health. There are so many things that go into this outcome, including our genetics. However, I am someone who likes to have a plan. I like to know what can affect my health in a negative way simply because I want to take action to the best of my ability, so I have the best chance to *remain in remission* and prevent future cancers.

When I look at my personal history and begin connecting the dots of risk factors, I begin to wonder how it didn't develop sooner!

Budget

Congratulations my friend! If you have read this far, then I know, without a shadow of a doubt, you are COMMITTED to your health. You are ready to do whatever it takes and you are searching for answers.

I'm sending you a massive hug through the book because that mentality is what will help you soar through this journey with flying colors.

I hope you have also gleaned through reading these chapters that there are many, many resources available to you. Which means there is at least *one* step you can take to further your health, regardless of your lifestyle, budget, or current treatment status.

This section is here to be mindful of those on a budget. If money isn't an issue, then throw money at your care! Hire every specialist you can, create your team, and rest in their knowledge and expertise. If you have *some* money then hire one specialist, and commit to their support and guidance. If you have a tight budget, then I would recommend using free, or low-cost information that is still valuable, like websites, podcasts, and books (see the resource chapter for all the recommendations). Then use whatever money you have available and put it towards the best nutrition and some supplementation to support your body as much as possible.

FREE resources would include:

- Blogs
- Podcasts
- Nutritional changes—start small and prioritize. Do what you can.

- Books. Even books can get pricey when you want to read 10-20! Get a library card and create a list of resource books you'd like to read.
- Online Health Summits. These are free if they are running live, otherwise it's a small investment to purchase later. Online health summits are collections of interviews, often videos or podcasts or both, on a certain topic.
- Leukemia and Lymphoma Society (www.lls.org). There are all sorts of patient resources, information, and support they provide to blood cancer patients. In fact, one service they offer is a $100 gift card for anyone diagnosed with blood cancer.
- Free dietitians or nutritional support at your treatment hospital (never hurts to ask and many hospitals are now including this type of service).
- Free classes or services at your treatment center which may include massage, essential oil classes, or fitness classes. Ask your doctor for a list of available resources.
- See the resource chapter for specific podcasts, books, free home cleaning services and more...

Small to medium investments:

- Going all organic in your diet
- Hiring a naturopath
- Working with a chiropractor/acupuncturist
- Hiring a nutritionist
- Getting regular massages. You may want to look for a certified oncology massage therapist
- Naturally Better With Cancer - an online program offered by Dr. Heather Paulson integrative oncologist
- Utilizing targeted supplements. If you can invest in ONE thing I would highly recommend hiring a naturopath who specializes in integrative cancer care to advise you on a supplement regimen while you go through treatment. Even if you are only

able to afford the one visit, you will learn something. If this is still out of range, then I would recommend following the advice in the book *Beating Cancer with Nutrition* and creating your own personal care plan from there.

- Online health summits (see above, if you have already gone through the free launch and now require purchase).

> Supplementation can have some of the most far-reaching impact of any steps you take in terms of mitigating (or preventing) side effects and keeping your body functioning well during treatment, so I cannot emphasize the importance I personally put on this. **If it's possible for you, this would be my NUMBER ONE investment recommendation, bar none.**

Large investments:

- Working regularly with an integrative oncologist/naturopath
- Working with or staying at a clinic (as part of, or after your conventional care)
- Therapists (conventional, biofeedback, emotional code therapy, or other)
- Specialists in any area that you may find supportive
- Detoxing your home and environment
- Other therapies like mistletoe, vitamin IV therapy, infrared sauna and more, (Only use these under guidance or recommendation of a practitioner. Many of these are only appropriate at certain stages during or after treatment.)

Wherever you are, I hope that this list brings you hope and encouragement. Small steps are still steps in the right direction. Remember, never compare your journey to anyone else's. *Your* life is unique and so is *your* healing journey.

12

Life after cancer

THE DAY I got my clear PET scan, I felt like such a schmuck. I knew that this should be super great, exciting, wonderful news! But for some reason I felt weird. Numb almost. I simply didn't know how to feel.

Part of what was happening was that for the past seven months I had to build this mental armor so that I could be strong and face what I needed to face. Then I got the clear PET, and while the cancer was gone, I discovered my tumor wasn't. That threw me a little bit and I think my mind was bouncing between: Do I celebrate? Can I take the armor off? Or do I still need to protect myself?

However you respond to news, good or bad, give yourself time. It took me about 24 hours to really process the information and begin to feel excited and get back to living as if I was cancer-free. It may take you longer, and that's ok too.

This new phase can be truly exciting. I know that the information in this book may give you a lot of homework as you dive into a new, healthy, nutrient-dense, toxin-free lifestyle. But whatever you do, don't allow it to overwhelm you. Start practicing ways to release stress and enjoy life. Take a vacation, go outside, visit family and splurge a little. Whatever you choose to do, don't live in fear.

Once it sunk in that I was cancer-free, I jumped right back in to "life". I started working more, writing this book, and getting back out there. But I had to realize that my body still needed time to recover.

I almost expected that as soon as I was cancer-free, my hair would be down to any shoulders again. Ha! But just like my hair is taking its grand old time growing back in, so your body needs time to get back to normal.

Once treatment is done, your body has a lot of work to do! Besides detoxing, which can take several years to do, your body has to get your hormones back into balance. It also has to rebuild your immune system and heal all the tissues, organs and microscopic traumas your body experienced during treatment!

You may notice that while you are progressively getting stronger and stronger, you still have bouts of fatigue, or that you have plenty of energy but for shorter durations of the day. This is all part of the process. The next few years will be interspersed with scans to make sure the tumor isn't growing and that everything is still ok. This is not the time to go back to bad habits, but rather, remission is the perfect time to continue investing time and energy back into your health!

My integrative oncologist and I are working on a step by step process to rebalance my hormones, and detox my body. So far, life just gets better and better! While I'd never wish this on anyone, I'm so thankful that I had this experience in order to share it with you.

If you'd like more support during your healing process, please reach out through my website www.kyleneterhune.com, or join my free Facebook group "Healthy Through Hodgkin's" where I share recipes, tips, and encouragement based on the topics in this book.

It is my sincere hope that this book brought you valuable information, resources, encouragement, and a realization that you are not alone.

There is a whole community of women out there just waiting to support and love you through this process, myself being one of them. I hope to connect soon to hear your story.

XOXO

Kylene

Books relating to cancer

- *Beating Cancer with Nutrition*, Patrick Quillin. Quillin worked with CTCA to design their nutrition recommendations and this is a textbook of information on navigating cancer and using nutrition to support your body while still getting conventional care.
- *Radical Remission*, Kelly A. Turner. An encouraging book about the common themes the author discovered when studying people who reverse their cancer and went into remission spontaneously.
- *The EBV Solution*, Kasia Kines. This is worth putting in here because EBV has been associated specifically with Hodgkin's and this is a textbook on what you can do to manage EBV which does not go away through chemotherapy. EBV is something that needs to be managed through life so that if you have a flare-up due to stress you are able to support your body and function well.
- *The Metabolic Approach to Cancer*, Dr. Nasha Winters
- *Chris Beat Cancer*, Chris Wark
- *Outside the Box Cancer Therapies*, Dr. Stengler and Dr. Anderson
- *Tripping over the Truth: How the metabolic theory of cancer is overturning one of medicine's most entrenched paradigms*, Travis Christofferson

Books about nutrition:

- *Wheat Belly*, Dr. William Davis. If you want to know more about why gluten is dangerous and should be avoided.
- *Beating Cancer with Nutrition*, Patrick Quillin. .Worked with CTCA to design their nutrition recommendations and this is a textbook of information on navigating cancer and using nutrition to support your body while still getting conventional care.

Other books:

- *The Christian Gratitude Journal*, Ben Greenfield www.kion.com
- *Earthing*, Clinton Ober

Blogs/Recipes:

- www.againstallgrain.com
- www.elanaspantry.com
- *The Cancer Fighting Kitchen*, Rebecca Katz
- *Green Smoothie Diet*, Robyn Openshaw

Alternative care or integrative clinics:

- Center for New Medicine, California
- Swiss Mountain Clinic, Switzerland
- The Paulson Clinic with Dr. Heather Paulson (Naturopathic integrative oncologist), Arizona, works virtually.
- The Center for Advanced Medicine with Dr. Jonathan Stegall (Integrative naturopath), Georgia www.tcfam.com
- The Bodhi Clinic, Maryland www.bodhiclinic.com
- Block Center for Integrative Cancer Care, Illinois www.block-md.com

Web page with a list of alternative care clinics:

www.cancure.org/10-list-of-clinics-in-the-united-states-offering-alternative-therapies/15-list-of-clinics-in-the-united-states-offering-alternative-therapies

Home cleaning products:

- Norwex: www.courtneyhemperly.norwex.biz

Laundry products:

- My Green Fills: www.mygreenfills.com
- Norwex: www.courtneyhemperly.norwex.biz

Skincare and Makeup:

- Beautycounter: www.beautycounter.com/KyleneT
- Crunchi: www.crunchi.com/stephaniellacuna

Air purifiers:

- www.airoasis.com
- www.hypoair.com

Water purifiers:

- The in home reverse osmosis unit we use: amzn.to/2JriKZ9\
- www.ispringwatersystems.com
- On counter: www.berkey.com/zestyginger
- www.aquatruwater.com
- Whole home: www.greenfieldnaturals.com

Shower filters:

- www.aquabliss.com

Home safety:

- www.HBELC.org
- www.Jibourenvironmental.com
- www.ehtrust.org
- www.createhealthyhomes.com
- www.greenbuildingsupply.com

Mold:

- www.zestyginger.com/moldy
- www.moldillnessmadesimple.com

EMF resources:

- Elana's Pantry: www.elanaspantry.com/wellness/?wellness-lifestyle=electromagnetic-field-emf
- Risa Suzuki: www.risasuzuki.com
- Dr. Mercola: www.articles.mercola.com/sites/articles/archive/2016/01/20/emf-controversy-exposed.aspx. He also has a book coming out in 2020: EMF*d.
- *Zapped: Why your cell phone shouldn't be your alarm clock*, Ann Louise Gittelman Radiation Nation - *a fallout of modern technology*, Daniel T. DeBaun and Ryan P. DeBaun

EMF blocking devices

- www.defendershield.com
- www.Ariestech.com
- www.shop.greensmoothiegirl.com/products/xzubi-disc

Cancer Podcasts:

- The Cancer Secrets Podcast, Dr. Stegall
- Ben Greenfield Podcast: Episodes *"Why you've been lied to about cancer and what you can do about it"* with Dr. Minkoff, and, *"The Mold-cancer link"* with Ian Clark.
- Take Control of Your Health podcast with Dr. Mercola: Episode *"Natural Cancer Therapies"* with Dr. Nasha Winters Anti-Cancer Revolution, Ryan Sternagel
- Chris Beat Cancer, Chris Wark

Other Health Podcasts:

- Lifelong Vitality with Kylene Terhune (that's me!!)
- The Model Health Show with Shawn Stevenson
- Broken Brain with Thru Purohit
- Wise Traditions with the Weston A Price Foundation
- The Functional Medicine Radio Show with Dr. Carri

Breast Cancer Resources
(because someday you can pay it forward!):

- Dr. Véronique Desaulniers DC: www.breastcancerconqueror.com
- Carol Lauri: www.ThePathofBreastCancer.com
- Breast Cancer Conqueror with Dr. V (Podcast)

Support after remission:

- www.ithriveplan.com (this is free to access)

Wigs/Scarves:

- Get a free scarf: www.goodwishesscarves.org/request-a-wrap/

- Get a free wig: hair.lovetoknow.com/
Free_Wigs_for_Cancer_Patients

Find resources available in your area:

www.cancer.org/treatment/support-programs-and-services/re-source-search.html

Simple Soul CBD. 25% off purchases for cancer patients. Register at the link below:

simplesoul.us/blog/simple-soul-cares?utm=kylene2

Sun Safety:

- Wise Traditions podcast #183 - *Is sunscreen okay to use?*
- *Embrace the Sun* by Marc Sorenson
- For chemical free sunscreen that is so clean you could eat it see: www.3rdrockessentials.com and use code TINYFITDIVA for a discount!
- www.safecosmetics.org

Random:

- Fluoride safety research and information: www.hiddencauseo-facne.com
- To protect from VOCs, chemicals and smells: www.Vogmask.com
- Online program "Naturally Better With Chemo" by Dr. Heather Paulson Integrative Oncologist
- 10 Questions to Ask Your Oncologist:
- https://kyleneterhunefdnp.lpages.co/
supplements-i-used-during-chemo

- 3 Things to Know when Diagnosed with Hodgkins
- https://kyleneterhunefdnp.lpages.
  co/3-things-to-know-when-diagnosed-with-hodgkins

For an updated list of resources, join the free **Healthy Through Hodgkins** Facebook group and click "files".

FIRST AND FOREMOST, I am nothing without my Savior. It has truly been in the darkest times that His light shines most brightly in my life. Without His infinite goodness, loving plans, and careful orchestration of events in my life, I would not be where I am today. I am thankful beyond measure that He chose to guide me down this path and use my life in this way.

To my loving husband Patrick. I cannot put into words what you mean to me. You are supportive and encouraging always. Without your support, I never would have become an FDN, gotten involved in functional health, and had the connections and opportunities that I have today. And without you, who would have run to the store a million times after treatment to pick up all the foods I was craving? I know that God chose you specifically as my best friend and partner for life and I love you forever.

To Keegan for being gentle and helpful when I was exhausted or feeling sick and bringing me anything I needed in bed. I love you more than you'll ever know, and I'm so proud to be your Mom.

To my parents. I know that this season has been stressful, but you smiled and trusted God the whole way. Thank you Dad for coming to every infusion and for being there for me. Thank you Mom for making delicious and spice-free meals the weekend after, and for sitting on my bed when I was exhausted and letting me blabber away. You are the best parents I could have been given and I love you both so much.

To my sisters who hung out with me, prayed for me, sent me gifts, and loved me.

To Dr. Heather Paulson for calming my fears, giving me amazing support, tools, and hope to navigate this journey and support my body in the best way possible. I know that the information and recommendations you gave me helped my body during and after treatment and that the way I feel now (AMAZING) is in large part thanks to YOU!

To CTCA and Dr. Redei for flying us out to Chicago, providing incredible patient care, offering a second option, staging, and answering all my questions. Thank you Dr. Redei for suggesting minimal treatment. It worked, and I'm grateful that my treatment time was cut in half because of you.

To my local oncologist. Thank you so much for being willing to look into things, try something new, and let me use my integrative approach and supplements. Thank you for being open and having a positive and kind demeanor. I was so glad you were my oncologist!

To each and every person, across the country, that was praying for me. There are too many of you to name, and many that I am not even aware of. Your prayers made a difference. Thank you.

To every friend, social media connection, or church member who took time out of their schedule to make me food, stop by, send a gift, write me a note, or make a care package. Those were bright spots during treatment and it meant so much to me that you would care enough to take the time. Thank you.

To my pathologist who was incredibly kind and considerate on a scary day filled with the unknown. Your sincerity, kindness, skill and attention to detail impacts lives in a positive way every day. Thank you.

To my editor Becky Alexander - you were the best. Thank you for your kind feedback, excellent skill, and communication through the process. You were a joy to work with!

To Outskirts Press for making this book possible and for a smooth ride the whole way through. You helped make my vision a reality!!

www.ingramcontent.com/pod-product-compliance
Lightning Source LLC
Chambersburg PA
CBHW051101250726
48656CB00001B/414